Concepts and Answers
for the MRCGP Oral Exam

Concepts and Answers for the MRCGP Oral Exam

P. Naidoo MBChB, MRCGP, DRCOG, Dip Occ Med, DFFP

GP in Oxfordshire

and

A. P. Davy MBBS, BSc, MRCGP, DRCOG

GP in the Defence Medical Services

Scion

© Scion Publishing Ltd, 2005

First published 2005

A CIP catalogue record for this book is available from the British Library.

ISBN 1 904842 06 2

Scion Publishing Limited
Bloxham Mill, Barford Road, Bloxham, Oxfordshire OX15 4FF
www.scionpublishing.com

Important Note from the Publisher
The information contained within this book was obtained by Scion Publishing Limited from sources believed by us to be reliable. However, while every effort has been made to ensure its accuracy, no responsibility for loss or injury whatsoever occasioned to any person acting or refraining from action as a result of information contained herein can be accepted by the authors or publishers.

The reader should remember that medicine is a contantly evolving science and while the authors and publishers have ensured that all dosages, applications and practices are based on current indications, there may be specific practices which differ between communities. You should always follow the guidelines laid down by the manufacturers of specific products and the relevant authorities in the country in which you are practising.

Production Editor: Clare Boomer
Typeset by Phoenix Photosetting, Chatham, Kent, UK
Printed by Biddles Ltd, Guildford, UK, www.biddles.co.uk

CONTENTS

CONCEPTS

MOCK QUESTIONS FOR EXAM PREPARATION

INDEX

PREFACE

The aim of this book is to help candidates prepare for the MRCGP oral examination, firstly by familiarising them with typical questions and answers, and secondly, by providing a structured approach to decision-making. The questions in the oral exam are designed to test the candidate's ability to make decisions, i.e.

- to recognise issues or dilemmas,
- select a defensible approach or viewpoint,
- explore the range of possible responses and,
- demonstrate an understanding of the principles that underpin their analysis of the problem posed.

Marks are awarded for the decision-making steps, not the final 'right' answer. This book provides a step-wise approach to decision-making. It also introduces various models and concepts which may be employed to generate a variety of perspectives so that a great many solutions can be offered.

P. Naidoo and A. Davy
January 2005

ACKNOWLEDGMENTS

I would like to thank Dr Helen Kingston for her inspirational teaching, Dr Samantha Wild, for being my very good friend and Dr Dougie Wyper for teaching me political incorrectness! Most of all, I would like to thank my husband Anton for believing in me.

Dr Prashini Naidoo

I would like to thank Pippa for inspiring me.

Dr Andrew P Davy

Both authors felt that the acknowledgments would be incomplete without mentioning Reitz and Jasper – thank you.

DEDICATION

This book is dedicated to our parents for giving us our sense of purpose and direction.

ABBREVIATIONS

BJGP	*British Journal of General Practice*
BMA	British Medical Association
BMJ	*British Medical Journal*
CAM	complementary and alternative medicine
CBT	cognitive behavioural therapy
CG	clinical governance
CHD	coronary heart disease
CHI	Commission for Health Improvement
CHRE	Council for Healthcare Regulatory Excellence
CME	continuing medical education
CPD	Continuing Professional Development
CPP	Committee on Professional Performance
DENs	doctors' educational needs
DVLA	Driver and Vehicle Licensing Agency
EBM	evidence-based medicine
GMC	General Medical Council
GP	general practitioner
GpwSI	GP with special interests
GUM	genito-urinary medicine
HFEA	Human Fertilisation and Embryology Authority
IUD	intra-uterine device
IVF	in vitro fertilisation
JAMA	*Journal of the American Medical Association*
JC	journal club
LCR	ligase chain reaction
MAAG	Medical Audit Advisory Group
MCA	Medical Council on Alcohol
MDU	medical defence union
MI	myocardial infarction
MUS	medically unexplained symptoms
NAPCE	National Association of Primary Care Educators
NCAA	National Clinical Assessment Authority
NEJM	*New England Journal of Medicine*
NHS	National Health Service
NICE	National Institute of Clinical Excellence
NNT	number needed to treat
NPSA	National Patient Safety Agency
OM	otitis media
PCC	Professional Conduct Committee
PCR	polymerase chain reaction
PCT	primary care trust
PDP	personal development plan
PHCT	Primary Health Care Trust

PID	pelvic inflammatory disease
PM	practice manager
PUNs	patients' unmet needs
RCGP	Royal College of General Practitioners
RCPCH	Royal College of Paediatrics and Child Health
RCT	randomised controlled trial
SEA	significant event audit
STD	sexually transmitted disease
UTI	urinary tract infection

INTRODUCTION

The oral module is one of the four modules comprising the MRCGP exam. The other three modules are:

- the written paper (Paper 1)
- the multiple choice paper (Paper 2)
- an assessment of consulting skills – either a videotape of the candidate's consultations or participation in a simulated surgery.

In this introductory chapter, we shall discuss:

- the structure of the exam
  - the structure of the MRCGP modular exam
  - the structure of the oral module
- the content of the oral module
- the marking of the oral exam
- preparing for the oral exam

THE STRUCTURE OF THE MRCGP EXAM

Modules can be taken at once or at different sessions. They can be taken in any order but all four must be passed. If candidates fail a module, they are allowed up to two further attempts; a fee is payable each time. The RCGP stipulates that all modules must be passed within three years of the application form being accepted otherwise all four modules must be retaken. Each of the four modules may be taken in the summer or the winter. The orals are held only in London and in Edinburgh.

THE STRUCTURE OF THE ORAL EXAM

Each candidate will be asked ten questions over a period of 40 minutes. The exam is divided into two 20-minute sessions. Each session is with a different pair of examiners. Each oral will consist of approximately five topics explored for about 4 minutes each. The examiners take it in turn to ask each topic. The exam can be disconcerting for a number of reasons:

- The examination hall is crowded. When candidates face their first set of examiners, they can see and hear the candidates sitting close by. It may take considerable effort to focus on the questions and not be distracted by the surrounding activity.
- The pace of the exam is brisk. The examiners need to get through ten questions in 40 minutes so they are fairly strict about moving on to the next question after 4 minutes. This may seem abrupt.
- Examiners may interrupt candidates and steer the questioning in different directions. This gives candidates the opportunity to move the discussion forward, so time is not wasted on topics that the candidate has already covered well and time is not wasted on areas of obvious deficiency.

- The examiners are not friendly GP trainers. Their job on the day is to test candidates and make decisions on grading. They tend not to help candidates along nor do they give non-verbal encouragement. Their poker faces can be quite intimidating. Some examiners are hawkish by nature and their rapidly-delivered questions and probing stares can be daunting.
- The exam questions are of varying difficulty. This allows the examiners to rank the candidates, to separate the pass/fail groups and to discriminate between the high-scoring and low-scoring candidates. There will be a few very difficult questions and within each question, each candidate will be pushed further along the decision-making process.
- Seven per cent of the candidates are video-recorded (with their consent). The video tapes are used for examiner training and do not form part of the candidates' assessment.

THE CONTENT OF THE ORAL EXAM

The aim of the oral exam is to test candidates' decision-making skills and their underpinning professional values and behaviour. Simpson (2004) proposed the adoption of a business model to aid the decision-making process. This model breaks decision-making into eight stages:

Table 1. *The business model for decision-making (Simpson, 2004)*
1. Recognise the dilemma
2. Identify possible options and solutions
3. Recognise the implications of these options
4. Prioritise and weigh each option
5. Choose an option
6. Justify choice
7. Check that the option works and does not need further modification or reassessment
8. Reflect on what has been learnt from the experience

Candidates score well if they:

- recognise the dilemma. Many of the problems require GPs to balance conflicting issues – for example, demand versus resources available, doing good as opposed to harm, the needs of the individual versus the needs of society.
- present a greater number of options together with the implications of each. Candidates should be able to discuss the advantages and disadvantages of each option – this demonstrates a deep understanding of the issue and shows the ability to anticipate the potential consequences of the decision.

Candidates must be prepared to justify why they dismissed some options as well as why they chose others.

Candidates should be able to make a decision. When pushed for a decision, candidates are expected to choose a plan of action and justify their choice. There is no textbook answer or college line to be regurgitated – examiners are looking for sound, ethical and evidence-based decision-making.

Candidates score well if they are able to construct an evaluation plan for the decision – in six months, how will they know that they made the correct decision?

The four examiners use a grid (see over) to place their topics in each of three 'Areas of Competence'. Each Area of Competence is then assessed in one of four contexts.

Examples of topics that have appeared in recent oral examinations are shown in the table overleaf.

WHAT THE MRCGP EXAM IS TESTING – MILLER'S PYRAMID

Miller (1990) proposed that one could assess skill at four levels of increasing sophistication:

1. knowledge (knows),
2. the ability to use that knowledge (knows how),
3. a demonstration that one can use that knowledge (shows how), and finally
4. the ability to use that knowledge in everyday practice (does).

The oral exam tests at level 3 – candidates must demonstrate to the examiner, by way of making decisions, their ability to use their knowledge.

- If the examiner wanted to test the candidates' knowledge of ethical principles, he could ask the candidate to list the components of an ethical framework. The candidate simply recalls what he has learnt.
- If he wanted to test the ability to apply knowledge, the examiner can provide a scenario, in the form of a modified essay question, to which the candidate must apply the ethical framework.
- If the examiner wants the candidate to *demonstrate* knowledge, then the candidate must overtly show a skill. A driving test demonstrates to the examiner the learner driver's skills – his ability to recognize problems on the road and to take appropriate action. Similarly, the oral exam tests the skills of decision-making and as in the driving test, the candidate must be overt in his demonstration of these skills. He has to show each step of the process – he does not jump to the conclusion. Marks are awarded for the steps, not the final 'right' answer.

	Communication	Professional values	Personal and professional growth
Care of patients	Breaking bad news Consultation models Verbal and non-verbal communication	Terminal care Ethics Medico-legal issues (consent and confidentiality)	Applying evidence-based medicine Clinical governance (audit, significant events, reflection) Managing change
Working with colleagues	Practice meetings Leadership and teamwork Employment issues (staff development and disciplinary actions)	Sick doctors Whistleblowing Transfer of patients between GP practices Extended scope of practice for nurses and community pharmacists Skills mix	Away days Staff appraisal Stress and burnout
Society	Communicating with the media Invitation to screening programmes/ health promotion	Rationing of care Euthanasia	Quality of care Professionalism (accountability, quality assurance, transparency)
Personal responsibility	'Heartsink' patients Removal of patients from lists Dealing with complaints	Gifts from patients Probity Sick notes	Revalidation Coping with uncertainty Mentoring Life-long learning and continued professional development

THE MARKING OF THE ORAL EXAM

Each examiner marks the question independently. A nine point scale is used – outstanding, excellent, good, satisfactory, bare pass, not adequate, unsatisfactory, poor and dreadful. Each mark is associated with a word picture, and the examiner's job is to decide which word picture best fits the candidate's response. At the end, the four examiners meet to collate their individual grades, with the overall mark being the aggregate of the four independent marks. If a candidate is on the pass/fail boundary, the examiners discuss the performance and make a judgement. The average pass rate for the oral examination during the three sessions from winter 2002 to summer 2004 has been approximately 83.4%.

PREPARING FOR THE ORAL EXAM

The RCGP's website advises candidates to prepare by maintaining 'a questioning and reflective approach to one's everyday work, regularly reviewing decisions taken – exploring alternative approaches, considering the wider implications of actions taken. Editorials in the *British Medical Journal* and the *British Journal of General Practice* are rich sources of debate on the important issues of our times.'

HOW TO READ AN EDITORIAL IN THE *BJGP* OR THE *BMJ*:

To understand a map, you need to be familiar with the key – you need to know what the different symbols on the map mean. Similarly, to understand editorials, review papers or policy documents, you need to have certain tools, which are listed below. After reading an editorial, write a summary using the template listed below (see *Table 2*).

- The concept – what main idea or theme is being discussed? Define the concept.
- The perspective – from what cultural, political or ethical perspective is it being discussed? What aspects of the discussion is the author emphasising and what is he downplaying?
- The theories or models – what explanation is being offered? What sequence of activities is being proposed to do something in a particular setting?
- What assumptions has the author made? What beliefs has he taken for granted? Is there any evidence to challenge or support the validity of these assumptions?
- Arguments are based on conclusions which are derived from claims to knowledge. The claim is made with varying degrees of certainty. Is there sufficient evidence to support the degree of certainty with which the claim was made?
- Evidence is usually derived from research that is done in a particular setting or context. Has the author 'generalised' the claim, i.e. moved it beyond its original context? Is there evidence to support the degree of generalisation in the claim being made?

Table 2. Template for summarising journal articles, adapted from Poulson and Wallace (2004)	
Authors Journal Type of article (editorial, theoretical paper, research paper, paper describing practice, policy paper)	
Concept discussed	
Perspective of discussion	
Theory/ model proposed	
Assumptions made	
Evidence to support certainty of claim	
Evidence to support generalisation of claim	

HOW BEST TO USE THIS BOOK

This book is divided into two parts:

1. The Questions and Answers section
2. The Concepts section

The Questions and Answers section will:

- pose a typical exam question.
- introduce the topic and tell you which area of the examiners' grid (see above) is being tested.
- use a model to generate a number of options, and discuss the advantages and disadvantages of each option.

The answer may go on to discuss the final decision taken by a typical candidate, as well as his or her justification for taking this stance, bearing in mind that the final decision should be based on a sound, ethical and evidence-based argument.

Background knowledge is required to:

- choose a model to generate the options – these may be consultation models, change management models or ethical frameworks.
- provide the evidence-base, where applicable, to justify the final decision.

The 'Additional information' section provides the background knowledge in greater detail. This is for candidates to reach a deeper understanding of the subject.

The 'Relevant literature' section signposts candidates to the primary sources of information. The literature changes at a rapid pace, and web sources are usually a good source of updated information, and so, where possible, useful websites are listed.

The Concepts section will:

- discuss common themes that run through most questions within the oral exam. The generic, background knowledge and skills that are required for the exam are discussed.

Alternative models for generating options are provided. This enables candidates to approach a question in the Questions and Answers section from an alternative perspective. Since high marks are awarded to candidates who are capable of generating a large number of options, it is important to consider multiple perspectives to an argument.

RELEVANT LITERATURE

Cottrell S (1999) **The study skills handbook.** Palgrave, Basingstoke.
Miller GE (1990) **The assessment of clinical skills/competence/performance.** *Academic Medicine*, **65,** 9 September, Supplement S63–7.
Poulson P and Wallace M (2004) **Learning to read critically in teaching and learning.** Sage, London.
Simpson RG (2004) **Preparing for the oral module.** *The Practitioner*, **248,** 287–289.
Royal College of General Practitioners MRCGP website: www.rcgp.org.uk/exam/

TO GET BEST RESULTS FROM THIS BOOK

- Read the introductory chapter.
- Skim through the concepts section, familiarising yourself with some models.
- Read the first five questions. After reading the questions, briefly answer them aloud or write down a 'construct' on a piece of paper. Read the answers provided and see if you could have added anything to your answers.

When you are revising for the second time:

- Read the 'Additional information' in the Questions and Answers section.
- Then read the relevant concepts chapters from the second half of the book. For the first five questions, these are the chapters on ethical frameworks and professionalism.
- Now read the questions again, and structure your answers using the business model for decision-making (see *Table 1* in the introductory chapter). Have you added anything new to your original answers?
- You can work though this process alone or you can generate answers in a group.

QUESTIONS AND ANSWERS

Care of the dying 1 (living wills):
76 year old Mr Jones has end-stage heart failure. He has been admitted to hospital six times in the past year with acute exacerbations. He comes to see you for advice on drawing up a living will. How would you advise Mr Jones? Discuss the possible advantages and disadvantages of advance directives.

This question tests the doctor's communication skills in the context of caring for patients.

We will use the *5 Ws and 1 H construct* to answer this question.

Definition of a living will
A living will, also called an advance directive, is a legally binding document drawn up in advance by a patient. It allows them to consent to or refuse specific medical treatments when they are too ill to communicate their decisions for themselves (BMA, 1995). Most people perceive advance directives as expressing a refusal of treatment. However, it may equally authorise that life-prolonging measures be maintained.

What does Mr Jones want?
Mr Jones can choose between six types of advance statements:

1. He can request the type(s) of treatment he would prefer in certain circumstances, e.g. if admitted with confusion, he would prefer not to have antibiotics.
2. He can state his general values and beliefs, e.g. he would prefer not to have a blood transfusion because he is a Jehovah's Witness.
3. He can name a proxy who knows him well enough that he or she can express the patient's wishes in the event of a life-threatening illness.
4. He can give instructions (directives) regarding his future treatment, e.g. he would prefer not to be admitted to the district hospital, but is happy to be treated at home or in the hospice.
5. He can specify that life-sustaining treatment can be withheld when he deteriorates irreversibly, e.g. if confused and restless, he would like to be made comfortable, but he would prefer not to have cardio-pulmonary resuscitation.
6. He can specify a combination of all the above.

Why would Mr Jones want a living will?
Mr Jones has certain values and beliefs which he would like expressed on his behalf during circumstances when he is unable to do so personally – he would like to protect his autonomy.

It is important to ensure that Mr Jones is not being coerced into making his declaration. Mr Jones may be tired, depressed and fed up with being 'put through the mill' with his numerous admissions. For a living will to be valid, the patient must be competent.

To meet the test of competence, Mr Jones must:

- comprehend and retain the necessary information,
- believe it,
- weigh up the information, balancing risks and needs, to arrive at a true choice.

If Mr Jones is depressed, then he is unlikely to believe the information regarding his treatment and thereby fails the test of competence (see chapter on ethical frameworks).

When would the living will come into existence?

Mr Jones needs to be given:

- adequate information regarding his treatments and
- time to make a reasoned judgement.

It is advisable that advance directives be drawn up with the aid of legal advice. Formatted versions are available from the Terence Higgins Trust or the Voluntary Euthanasia Society. The directive should contain the following check-list:

- Mr Jones' full name and address
- Name and address of his own GP
- The date on which the document was drawn up
- The date on which the document will be reviewed (usually when circumstances change or in five years)
- A statement indicating that advice was obtained from health professionals
- A clear statement of the patient's wishes
- The contact details of the nominated proxy.

Once completed, the living will should be witnessed and signed by the patient, their GP, their solicitor and the nominated proxy.

Who is the proxy?

Mr Jones' proxy (or surrogate) will have continuing power of attorney. He or she should be emotionally stable and should be able to make reasoned judgements based on adequate information in the patient's best interests.

Where are the documents kept?

A copy should be kept by the patient, his solicitor, his GP and his hospital. Mr Jones could also wear a medic-alert bracelet so that the emergency services are also informed.

How would the doctor advise Mr Jones?

Advice would be based on the following questions:

- Is Mr Jones mentally competent at presentation?
- Has the GP given Mr Jones adequate information so that he can make an informed decision – has he understood the consequences of his decisions?
- Is he being coerced?
- Has he nominated a proxy?

- Has he decided which directives he would like to exercise (see list of six choices)
- Has he informed his family, his proxy and his solicitor?
- Is the document correctly drawn up? See above check-list.

Discuss the possible advantages and disadvantages of advance directives.

ADVANTAGES

- The patient's autonomy is recognised and respected. This is reassuring to the patient.
- Everybody is made aware in advance of the patient's wishes. The advance directive may reduce confusion arising during stressful situations.
- It provides relief to family and friends by unburdening them from the difficult decisions regarding treatment.

DISADVANTAGES

- Patients may change their minds when actually confronted by reality – their perspective may change as their health declines.
- The living wills may lack sufficient information – they are left open to interpretation.
- The living wills may be too specific – they may not cover every eventuality.
- Patients cannot refuse basic care – hygiene, pain relief and the offer of oral nutrition and hydration.
- Various health care professionals may look after the patient – many of them may be unaware of the document's existence. Surveys show that only 49% of GPs knew that advance directives were legally binding and only 25% of hospital trusts had policies for them (RCP, 1998).
- Relatives may be distressed if previously unaware of the living will's existence.

LEARNING POINTS

- Advance directives are legally binding
- Test of competence
- Terence Higgins Trust or the Voluntary Euthanasia Society
- Patients cannot refuse basic care

ADDITIONAL INFORMATION

Michael Jarmulowicz, consultant histopathologist, Royal Free Hospital wrote a response to Diggory P and Judd M (2000) Advance directives: questionnaire survey of NHS trusts. *BMJ*, **320**, 24–5.

'The medical profession has moved from a paternalistic position of "doctor knows best" to one in which the patient gives informed consent. For consent to be valid the patient must understand both the expected benefits of the proposed treatment and the possible adverse consequences. If informed consent for treatment is right, then it is equally right, both morally and logically, that refusal of treatment should be equally informed. But informed refusal of treatment can be valid only if the specific facts pertaining to the current situation are available. It is likely that living wills will be made many years prior to mental incompetence, when details of the conditions specified – including possible treatments available – cannot be foreseen.

In many scenarios a legally binding living will could bring about the distressing situation that the testator was trying to avoid. For example, a patient may state that surgery must not be performed if terminal cancer is present, but palliative surgery may be indicated in terminal bowel cancer, not to prolong life, but to relieve the distressing symptoms associated with unrelieved bowel obstruction. In such a case a legally binding "living will" will prohibit doctors from providing the most appropriate palliative care available.'

Emanuel LL *et al.* (1991) Advance directives for medical care – a case for greater use. *NEJM*, **324,** 889–895.

This study investigated the attitudes of patients toward advance directives in an outpatient setting in Boston, USA.

The study concluded that when people are asked to imagine themselves incompetent with a poor prognosis, they decide against life-sustaining treatments about 70 percent of the time. Health, age, or other demographic features cannot be used, however, to predict specific preferences. Advance directives as part of a comprehensive approach such as that provided by the Medical Directive are desired by most people, require physician initiative, and can be achieved during a regular office visit.

Consent

For consent to be valid,

- the patient must be sufficiently informed;
- the patient must be competent; and
- consent must be given voluntarily.

What patients ought to know (from *Seeking patients' consent: the ethical considerations*, General Medical Council, November 1998)

The information which patients want or ought to know, before deciding whether to consent to treatment or an investigation, may include:

- details of the diagnosis, and prognosis, and the likely prognosis if the condition is left untreated;
- uncertainties about the diagnosis including options for further investigation prior to treatment;

- options for treatment or management of the condition, including the option not to treat;
- the purpose of a proposed investigation or treatment; details of the procedures or therapies involved, including subsidiary treatment such as methods of pain relief; how the patient should prepare for the procedure; and details of what the patient might experience during or after the procedure including common and serious side effects;
- for each option, explanations of the likely benefits and the probabilities of success; and discussion of any serious or frequently occurring risks, and of any lifestyle changes which may be caused by, or necessitated by, the treatment;
- advice about whether a proposed treatment is experimental;
- how and when the patient's condition and any side effects will be monitored or re-assessed;
- the name of the doctor who will have overall responsibility for the treatment and, where appropriate, names of the senior members of his or her team;
- whether doctors in training will be involved, and the extent to which students may be involved in an investigation or treatment;
- a reminder that patients can change their minds about a decision at any time;
- a reminder that patients have a right to seek a second opinion;
- where applicable, details of costs or charges which the patient may have to meet.

Kirk P, Kirk I *et al.* (2004) What do patients receiving palliative care for cancer and their families want to be told?: a Canadian and Australian qualitative study. *BMJ*, **28**(7452), 1343–7.

72 participants registered with palliative care were interviewed.

- The study found that the process of sharing information is as important as the content. The timing, management, and delivery of information and perceived attitude of practitioners were critical to the process. This applied to information interactions at all stages of the illness.
- Main content areas mentioned related to prognosis and hope. Hope can be conveyed in different ways.
- Secondary information from various sources is accessed and synthesised with the primary information.
- All patients, regardless of origin, wanted information about their illness and wanted it fully shared with relatives.
- Almost all patients requested prognostic information, and all family members respected their wishes.
- Information was perceived as important for patient–family communication. Information needs of patient and family changed and diverged as illness progressed, and communication between them became less verbally explicit.

The study concluded that information delivery for patients needs to be individualised with particular attention to process at all stages of illness. Patients and families use secondary sources of information to complement and verify information given by health carers.

RELEVANT LITERATURE

Advance directives in the UK: legal, ethical, and practical considerations for doctors. *BJGP* 1998, **48,** 1263–6 (May).

BMA (1995) **Advance statements about medical treatment – code of practice report of the BMA.**

BMA (1999) **Withholding and withdrawing life-prolonging treatment.**

Best practice is outlined in an easy-to-read Australian document entitled **'Using advance care directives':** http://www.health.nsw.gov.au/pubs/2004/pdf/adcare_directive.pdf

GMC (2002) Withholding and withdrawing life-prolonging treatments. Good practice in decision-making. www.gmc-uk.org

GMC (1998) **Seeking patients' consent: the ethical considerations.** www.gmc-uk.org

A very good summary on advance directives is available from the British Geriatrics Society website: http://www.bgs.org.uk/compendium/compg2.htm

RCP (1998) **Do general practitioners know when living wills are legal? 32,** 351–353.

Care of the dying 2 (withholding life-prolonging treatment):
77 year old Mr Jones with end-stage heart failure saw you a year ago to draw up a living will stating that he did not want to be admitted to hospital or be given life-saving treatment in the event of irreversible deterioration. A few months ago he suffered a stroke and is now demented and bed-bound. His wife, who cares for him at home, requests a visit. After examining him, you suspect that he has pneumonia. His devoted wife, who is also his proxy, wants you to prescribe antibiotics. What would you do?

This question tests the doctor's communication skills in the context of caring for patients. It also tests a doctor's professional values in the context of society's changing attitudes and expectations.

An ethical framework may be applied to the above scenario. The moral dilemma in this situation is maintaining a respect for the patient's autonomy on the one hand, or treating him in his best interests on the other.

AUTONOMY

A living will is a legally binding document that expresses the patient's autonomy. It is valid if:

- Mr Jones was competent at the time the decisions were made.
- he was given sufficient information to understand the consequences of his choices.
- he was not coerced into making the advance directive.
- the directive is applicable to his current situation.

Mr Jones drew up the directive after a series of hospital admissions with acute exacerbations of heart failure. The directive states he did not want admission to hospital and he would prefer that life-sustaining treatment be withheld should he deteriorate irreversibly.

- Would Mr Jones want to be kept alive in his current bed-bound demented state?
- Would he have considered his current state to be a burden on his family?
- Is the directive too vague? By life-sustaining treatment, was Mr Jones referring to cardio-pulmonary resuscitation as well as antibiotics?

BENEFICENCE

The doctor would want to act in the patient's best interests. Giving Mr Jones antibiotics would prevent pain and suffering – they may be regarded as palliative rather than life-saving. What would the doctor do if Mrs Jones wanted him to have a course of antibiotics at home?

The GMC advises that the doctor takes the following factors into account when deciding which treatment is in the patient's best interests:

- Is the treatment clinically indicated? In this case, pneumonia is a clear indication for giving antibiotics.
- Is there any evidence of an advance directive or does the doctor know what the patient would have wanted? Unfortunately the living will in this case lacks sufficient information and is left open to interpretation. Mrs Jones may not consider antibiotics to be 'life-saving' in the same way as CPR or ventilation in ITU.
- What are the views of the close family? Does the Jones family want to give the patient antibiotics and not see this form of treatment as a breach of his advance directive?
- If there are a few treatment options, choose the option that least restricts the patient's future choices. In the case of Mr Jones, there are two reasonable options: to give or not to give, but not to give is more likely to result in his death, thus restricting his future choices.

NON-MALEFICENCE

First do no harm. Oral antibiotics may be given and they may have very few side effects. They could prevent overwhelming infection and a potentially distressing death. The potential good and harm of the therapeutic intervention needs to be weighed up to decide what overall is in the patient's best interests.

Summary of case

The doctor should talk to Mrs Jones, who is both wife and proxy, to clarify her reasons for wanting antibiotics. If other relatives are present, the doctor should reach a consensus on whether to give antibiotics. A dilemma arises if the doctor feels that he is not respecting Mr Jones' autonomy by giving antibiotics and Mrs Jones feels that the doctor is not acting in her husband's best interests by withholding treatment. Are the other close family members aware of what Mr Jones would have wanted? The doctor could speak to other health professionals, such as the district nurses, to get their opinions. What quality of life would he have if he survived this episode? Discussions and decisions reached should be well documented. If resolution is difficult, the GP could get advice from a consultant in elderly care and his medical defence union.

What would you do?

I would give antibiotics because:

- The advance directive is not specific enough. Mr Jones may not have considered antibiotics to be a life-saving treatment in the same way that CPR and ventilation are.
- His wife, who is also his proxy, is making a reasonable request for oral antibiotics to prevent unnecessary suffering. Her views need to be respected. If not, she can accuse the GP of negligence.
- The benefits of antibiotics outweigh the possible harms.

- The doctor would be acting in the spirit of the GMC guidance on treating in a patient's best interests. It states that the option which least restricts the patient's future choice should be chosen.

I would not give antibiotics because:

- I know the patient well and would therefore be respecting his values and beliefs by not prolonging his life with antibiotics.
- His quality of life is poor. In accordance with palliative care philosophy, I would ensure that he is pain-free and comfortable and I would allow him to die with dignity.
- If conflict arises between Mrs Jones and myself, I could apply to the courts for a decision.

LEARNING POINTS

- Determinants of the validity of an advance directive
- The patient's 'best interests'
- The conflict between 'autonomy' and 'best interests'

ADDITIONAL INFORMATION

The following advice is taken from: **GMC (2002)** *Withholding and withdrawing life-prolonging treatments: good practice in decision-making.* **See:** http://www.gmc-uk.org/standards/whwd.htm

Adult patients who cannot decide for themselves

1. Any valid advance refusal of treatment – one made when the patient was competent and on the basis of adequate information about the implications of his/her choice – is legally binding and must be respected where it is clearly applicable to the patient's present circumstances and where there is no reason to believe that the patient had changed his/her mind.

2. Where adult patients lack capacity to decide for themselves, an assessment of the benefits, burdens and risks, and the acceptability of proposed treatment must be made on their behalf by the doctor, taking account of their wishes, where they are known. Where a patient's wishes are not known it is the doctor's responsibility to decide what is in the patient's best interests. However, this cannot be done effectively without information about the patient which those close to the patient will be best placed to know. Doctors practising in Scotland need additionally to take account of the Scottish legal framework for making decisions on behalf of adults with incapacity.

Care of the dying 3 (euthanasia):

Mr Jones is given oral antibiotics at home. Unfortunately he continues to deteriorate. His wife is increasingly distressed by his loud, raspy breathing. She asks you to give him a large dose of morphine. How would you react?

This question tests the doctor's professional values in the context of caring for patients while being sensitive to society's changing attitudes and expectations.

Doctors are legally bound not to assist suicide or take any action of which the primary purpose is to end life. However, the double-effect doctrine holds: a doctor can administer a dose of painkiller if the primary aim is to relieve pain, even if the secondary effect is to shorten the patient's life.

A consultation model can be used to navigate the potential minefield of the above scenario. I will use Berne's model of transactional analysis which looks at the roles that patients and doctors play within the consultation (Berne, 1968). Berne identifies three ego states:

- Parent: may be critical or caring. In this mode, the doctor or patient commands, directs, prohibits, controls and/or nurtures the other party.
- Adult: The doctor or patient sorts out information and works logically.
- Child: The doctor or patient assumes the dependent role.

When doctors are asked to assist in a patient's death, they should explore the reasons behind the request in an adult–adult fashion:

- What is Mrs Jones really asking for – is she indicating that she believes her husband to be in pain? Is better symptom control required?
- Is Mrs Jones indicating that she cannot cope with his care any more and she would prefer that he be cared for in a hospice or hospital?
- Is Mrs Jones acting in accordance with her husband's wishes – did he hope to avoid a long, drawn-out death?
- Is Mrs Jones grief-stricken and depressed? Is she expressing her feelings of hopelessness?

By thinking through what the problem really is, both Mrs Jones and the doctor are sorting out the information logically (adult–adult relationship). They come to a shared understanding of the problem and negotiate a course of action that is respectful of each other's views. The GP should explain what is and is not legally acceptable. In the UK, assisted suicide is currently illegal. However, a doctor should acknowledge the legitimacy of the request and express empathy for her situation.

The consultation is in danger of becoming a parent–child discussion when the doctor either reacts in a critical manner 'How could you put me in this position?' or in a directive manner 'Let me call the palliative care services and we'll sort it out for you!'

The consultation is in danger of becoming a child–parent discussion when the doctor abandons his professional judgement in an attempt to please Mrs Jones.

Talking to Mrs Jones is fundamental to understanding her concerns, reassuring her and maintaining the doctor–patient relationship. Mrs Jones may require further support from a psychiatric nurse or a spiritual adviser.

Mr Jones has not been able to eat for the past four days. The district nurse asks if she should start nasogastric fluids and feeds. Nutrition and hydration are a medical treatment that a competent patient may refuse. Mr Jones is incompetent, but his previously expressed wishes and those of his family should be taken into account. The dilemma arises as some doctors consider fluid and feeds to be basic necessities while others consider them to be medical treatments.

Mr Jones deteriorates a day into your fortnight's annual leave. You are the only doctor to have seen him in the last fourteen days. Your partner is called to confirm death. Mrs Jones wants her husband cremated. What should your partner do?

Your partner should visit Mr Jones to examine the body and confirm death. He should then discuss the case with the coroner. He can sign the death certificate, but the certificate asks when the patient was last seen by the signing doctor. Even if he hadn't attended in the last fourteen days, he can sign if he had seen the patient previously. This is the date which must be noted.

Cremation cannot occur until the cause of death has been established and the coroner rules that a post-mortem is not needed. The following forms are required:

- The next of kin signs the cremation application form.
- Section B is completed by the doctor who issued the death certificate.
- Section C is completed by a doctor who is not related to, or in practice with, the first doctor.
- The Register of Deaths issues the certificate of disposal (green form).

LEARNING POINTS

- Berne's model of transactional analysis
- Death certification
- Cremation forms
- Euthanasia: arguments for and against

ADDITIONAL INFORMATION

Morritt AN and Hall J (2004) Completing a death certificate. *BMJ Career Focus*, **328**(7451), 217–217.

Filling in the death certificate:

- Part 1a: state the disease or pathological disorder leading to death – for example, myocardial infarction. It is not the mode of dying – for example, cardiac arrest.
- Parts 1b and 1c: state diseases underlying part 1a – for example, ischaemic heart disease.
- Part 2: state diseases that may have contributed to the death but were not part of the main causal sequence – for example, dementia.

Also see: http://www.medicalprotection.org/medical/united_kingdom/publications/: GPs typically attend fewer deaths than hospital doctors – perhaps 5 each year. An average GP list will see around 25 deaths a year, most of which will be in hospital.

Deaths which require further investigation are reported to the local coroner. The coroner decides whether to arrange a post-mortem and/or hold an inquest.

There are therefore three categories of death (figures for England and Wales in 2001 are given for each):

- certified by a doctor (332 000 – 62%);
- certified by a doctor after authorisation by a coroner (79 000 – 15%); and
- certified by a coroner (122 000 – 23%).

The following advice is taken from: GMC (2002) *Withholding and withdrawing life-prolonging treatments: good practice in decision-making.* **See:** http://www.gmc-uk.org/standards/whwd.htm

Artificial nutrition and hydration

Where death is imminent, in judging the benefits, burdens or risks, it usually would not be appropriate to start either artificial hydration or nutrition, although artificial hydration provided by the less invasive measures may be appropriate where it is considered that this would be likely to provide symptom relief.

Where death is imminent and artificial hydration and/or nutrition are already in use, it may be appropriate to withdraw them if it is considered that the burdens outweigh the possible benefits to the patient.

Where death is not imminent, it usually will be appropriate to provide artificial nutrition or hydration. However, circumstances may arise where you judge that a patient's condition is so severe, and the prognosis so poor that providing artificial nutrition or hydration may cause suffering, or be too burdensome in relation to the possible benefits. In these circumstances, as well as consulting the health care team and those close to the patient, you must seek a second or expert opinion from a senior clinician (who might be from another discipline such as nursing) who has experience of the patient's condition and who is not already directly involved in the patient's care. This will ensure that, in a decision of such sensitivity, the patient's interests have been thoroughly considered, and will provide necessary reassurance to those close to the patient and to the wider public.

Euthanasia

Arguments against:
- The killing of innocent human beings is morally wrong. The sanctity of human life is embodied in most religious teachings.
- The current system for treating terminally ill patients provides humane palliative care. Most forms of pain can be controlled. Where alternatives exist, there is no need for euthanasia.
- Changing the legislation may be dangerous because of the abuse that may occur.

- Elderly patients may become fearful of seeking medical attention in case their relatives and doctors choose euthanasia when they become incompetent. The cost of looking after terminally ill patients is increasing. On discharge from hospital, patients may need extensive care from the family or admission to a nursing home – this may place a financial burden on the family.
- People may feel pressurised into accepting euthanasia so as not to burden their relatives.

Arguments for:
- Individuals should have the right to choose the manner and timing of their death.
- Euthanasia would prevent people dying in pain and distress.
- Everyone should be able to die with dignity.

Ethics

When moral dilemmas occur in the context of caring for terminally ill patients, the following ethical concepts need to be considered:

- Relativism – the idea that there are no absolute rights or wrongs – the morality of any action depends on the circumstances or culture.
- Doctrine of double-effect – an action that has both good and bad effects may be justifiable (e.g. administering opiates in terminal care).
- Ordinary and extraordinary means – some treatments may not be justifiable because of the degree of intervention required (e.g. antibiotics for an infection in end-stage respiratory failure may be justified, but ventilation may not be).
- Futility – if an outcome is going to be poor anyway, any intervention or treatment needs to be judged in this light.
- Wants and needs – fair resource allocation demands an objective assessment of needs. How can this be done?

RELEVANT LITERATURE

See http://www.mja.com.au/public/issues/181_08_181004/ash10074_fm.html for a very good summary on the ethics and legality of artificial nutrition and hydration to patients in a persistent vegetative state.
See http://www.parliament.uk/parliamentary_committees/lordsassisted.cfm for details of the evidence provided in November 2004 to The Lords' Committee which was set up to scrutinise the *Assisted Dying for the Terminally Ill Bill*. Evidence was presented by the Department of Health, Royal Society of Psychiatrists and the Disability Rights Commission.

This question tests the doctor's communication skills in the context of caring for patients.

I would apply a consultation model to answer the above question. Helman's folk model of illness (1981) attempts to answer the following questions:

- What has happened?
- Why has it happened?
- Why to me?
- Why now?
- What would happen if nothing were done about it?
- What should I do about it?

Patients construct in their minds an idea or explanation of what is happening to them based on their experiences, imagination and peer group views. Therefore Helman's folk model of illness is a useful tool for understanding a patient's ideas, concerns and expectations, particularly during challenging life experiences.

WHAT HAS HAPPENED?

Mr Patel has lost his young wife and is now left with two young children to care for. He may have practical, financial, and emotional demands to meet. He may or may not have a support network that he can access. He may be seeing you for a variety of reasons – it is important not to presume to know his feelings and reasons for attending and to explicitly clarify his agenda. Is Mr Patel seeing you to discuss

- emotional issues – after all, he is crying in your consulting room. Has he been able to express his grief in public or has he maintained a 'stiff upper lip' for his children and wider family?
- practical and financial issues – Mr Patel may be finding it difficult to balance his home life and work life. Child-care arrangements or custody battles may be distressing him. He may need signposting to Social Services and support networks.

Freud wrote that grief is a normal reaction to the loss of a loved one and that grieving is a painful process involving the withdrawal of ties to the deceased. The main task of grieving is to detach yourself from the emotional ties to the deceased so that new relationships can be formed.

Traditional models of grief (initial shock, yearning, despair and recovery) were based chiefly on the work of Kübler-Ross (1969). They have been replaced by more recent models that suggest grief reactions are not stepwise – there are swings in mood, thoughts and behaviour.

WHY HAS IT HAPPENED?

What mental construct has Mr Patel made of the experience? Is he a fatalist and believes that Helen's death was part of a divine plan? Is he angry with God, his wife or the medical profession?

WHY TO ME?

Mr Patel's explanation of why the event has occurred tells us about his *'locus of control'*:

- An internal controller is someone who believes that he is in charge of his health.
- An external controller believes that a divine presence is in control of his health – a fatalist.
- Some people believe in 'the powerful other' and see doctors as being in control of their health.

WHY NOW?

Mr Patel may have certain religious or cultural views about why the death has occurred now and these may be in conflict with those of Helen's family. He may find it difficult to reconcile these views.

WHAT WOULD HAPPEN IF NOTHING WERE DONE ABOUT IT?

Mr Patel may be exhibiting a normal grief reaction or his emotional distress may be affecting his ability to function adequately at home or at work. In Western society, grief is a taboo subject – friends and relatives may not know what to say and be avoiding Mr Patel. Perhaps he is being advised to 'keep busy and get on with it' and may be in danger of becoming isolated. There are cultural differences in reactions to bereavement: in Western society, reminders of the deceased are discouraged whereas in traditional Hindu society, photographs of the deceased are often displayed in a shrine.

Being male and having poor social support are risk factors for poor outcome after bereavement.

WHAT SHOULD I DO ABOUT IT?

Mr Patel may simply need support and understanding. Support from a charity may also be helpful (CRUSE: www.cruse-bereavementcare.org.uk). Occasionally, bereavement counselling and treatment for depression are indicated.

ADDITIONAL INFORMATION

Practice should have procedures in place to assist bereaved patients.

- A practice leaflet to inform patients what to do at the time of death could be useful.
- Usually patients die in the hospital. The surgery should contact the nearest relative by personalised letter, by visiting or by telephone. Relatives are often grateful for this offer of support.
- The date of bereavement should be recorded in the nearest relative's notes as anniversaries can be difficult times.

Zarit SH (2004) Family care and burden at the end of life (editorial). *Canadian Medical Association Journal*, **170**(12), 1811–2.

Family members provide a considerable amount of the care for people with terminal illnesses and their own health may suffer as a consequence. A study of 89 caregivers of women with advanced breast cancer showed that:

- caregivers were significantly more anxious than patients and
- were substantially more likely to be depressed.
- the caregivers reported a considerable increase in burden and depression by the time the patients reached the terminal stage of illness.
- over three-quarters of those who were employed reported that they had to miss work because of their caregiving responsibilities.

RELEVANT LITERATURE

Helman CG (1981) **Diseases versus illness in General Practice.** *Journal of Royal College of General Practitioners.* **31,** 548–52.
Kübler-Ross E (1969) **On death and dying.** *Springer*, New York.
Parkes CM (1989) **Bereavement in adult life.** *BMJ*, **316,** 856–859.
Sheldon F (1998) **ABC of palliative care: bereavement.** *BMJ*, **316,** 465–458.

This question tests the doctor's professional values in the context of interacting with society. A doctor can be considered to be 'good' by his patients, his profession, his colleagues and his family.

PROFESSIONAL QUALITIES

A good doctor follows the profession's code of practice, as laid down by the GMC in *Good medical practice* (2001). The doctor makes his patients his first concern and is respectful of the patients' primacy. The doctor is honest, trustworthy and ethical. He maintains his patients' confidentiality and establishes a relationship that is based on trust. He obtains appropriate informed consent and decides on treatments that are in his patients' best interests. The doctor does not abuse his position in society. He maintains his financial and personal integrity (probity). A good doctor is also a safe doctor – he recognises the limits of his competence and does not put his patients at risk. He continues to improve his knowledge, skills, attitudes and professional values – he actively learns from his work and keeps up to date. He does not engage in unethical research.

PERSONAL QUALITIES

- Caritas – the Latin word *caritas* describes the qualities of genuine caring that the doctor has for his patients. Good doctors are sensitive, empathetic, understanding, patient-centred and approachable.
- Self-awareness – a good doctor has insight into his own motives, needs and feelings. He is able to ask for help. He is able to challenge his assumptions and knowledge without being defensive and resistant to change.
- Good interpersonal skills – he is able to contribute to and appreciate the value of team work. He demonstrates leadership skills and is able to support other members of the group.
- He has good communication skills – he is able to listen and respond appropriately. He analyses well, marshals his facts, argues a case and establishes priorities.
- He has a good sense of humour, is conscientious, tolerant, flexible and affable.
- He is motivated, enthusiastic and committed to his work.
- He is able to achieve a good balance between his professional and private life. He is personally well organised and able to set good boundaries.

Leader and team player
He listens to and respects the views of all team members. He is skilled at motivating the quieter members of the team to contribute and skilfully moderates the more voluble. He is a skilled negotiator who provides a clear and detailed

vision of what the team requires and encourages team members to work towards these goals.

What society expects

Society expects doctors to keep the patient at the focus of the consultation, to put the needs of the patient first, to be patient-centred. Doctors can achieve patient-centredness by:

- reducing sapiential authority. Sapiential authority is possessed by virtue of the person's special knowledge, expertise and experience. Historically, the authority of doctors grew because they knew more about disease and treatments than did their patients. Patients did not question the doctors and doctors rarely admitted that they did not know the answers. Doctors can reduce their sapiential authority by facilitating their patients' access to information, by explaining the treatment options in simple language and allowing patients to make the choice that suits them best.
- reducing moral authority. Moral authority is possessed by virtue of the person's concern for the afflicted individual. Society expects doctors to work in the best interests of their patients. In the aftermath of the Bristol scandal and the Shipman murders, public confidence in the 'inherent good' of doctors has waned. Clinical governance, with its emphasis on transparency, accountability, and cultural openness is perhaps an attempt by the profession to show society that doctors are acting in the patients' best interests rather than in their own.
- reducing charismatic authority. Charismatic authority is possessed by virtue of the afflicted person's faith that the doctor will be of help. A doctor was seen as having the healing power that was given by God to a chosen individual. There is a general social trend towards informality and openness. The priestly white coat has disappeared from general practice. Patients are more questioning of their doctors.

RELEVANT LITERATURE

Neighbour R (1992) **The inner apprentice.** *Kluwer Academic Publishers*, Newbury, UK.
Tate P (2002) **The doctor's communication handbook.** *Radcliffe Medical Press*, Oxford.
www.resourcefulpatient.org/ by Dr Muir Gray and Dr Harry Rutter.

This question tests the doctor's personal and professional growth in the context of patient care and/or working with colleagues. This question can also be phrased as 'how do you identify your learning needs?' or 'how do you keep up to date?'

There are five stages to the continuing professional development (CPD) cycle:

- Assessment of individual and organisational needs
- Making personal development plans
- Implementation
- Reinforcement and dissemination
- Review of the effectiveness of the CPD intervention

AN ASSESSMENT OF LEARNING NEEDS

Learning needs can be conceptualised as the discrepancy between the starting point ('where are you now?') and the end point ('where do you want to be?') (Kaufman, 1979).

Learning needs can be identified from personal review, clinical practice, from patients and from colleagues with whom you work.

From personal review
- Personal reading, internet and media, lectures and meetings, further study (e.g. diplomas) and research.
- Formal testing, e.g. quizzes in medical magazines; PEP-CDs; *BMJ*-learning modules; SWOT-analysis where the doctor identifies the strengths and weaknesses of his practice and the opportunities and threats to his progress; and Manchester Rating Scales.
- Reflection on challenging consultations or interactions (what happened?; why did it happen?; what can I do differently next time to alter the outcome?).
- Videos of consultations / joint surgeries: actual performance is reviewed by the doctor or by a peer to see if the desired behaviours are present, e.g. did the doctor demonstrate empathy?

From clinical practice
- Audits: Audit is a measurement of quality. It compares the actual level of performance against clearly defined, explicit standards. Changes are made and their effect is re-measured to see if they had the desired outcome. There should be self-improvement through standard setting, measurement, change and reassessment.
- MAAG audits (Medical Audit Advisory Group): compares the performance of the practice with other local practices; prioritises areas of clinical practice that need improvement (e.g. diabetic care); and shares ideas for improvement.

- Significant event analysis (SEA): is a review of critical or important events. It includes positive and negative events. The team reviews the strengths and weaknesses of the management and identifies ways in which things could be done differently. The aim is for the entire team to learn from the event and to apply the lessons learnt.
- Feedback from patient groups: the groups' views are incorporated in the practice plan.

From patients
- PUNs and DENs (patients' unmet needs and doctors' educational needs). Patients may ask doctors questions to which they do not know the answer. Doctors have to find the answer, so meeting their educational needs.
- Complaints.
- Patient satisfaction surveys and questionnaires: In addition to providing feedback on their overall experience of the practice, they also comment on the doctor's timekeeping and attitudes. The Royal College of General Practitioners advises that patient surveys be done on an annual basis.

From the team
- Staff feedback: either informally through practice meetings or formally through 360° feedback. 360° feedback involves handing out a questionnaire to a cross-section of the PHCT (everyone from receptionist to senior partner). The information is collected anonymously by a third party who analyses and feeds back to the individual so that he becomes aware of how others see him – Johari's window.
- Practice appraisals: The practice may be inspected by the PCT, the Committee for Health Improvement, and the deanery (if it is a training practice).
- PACT: prescribing trends within the practice compared to others regionally.

From other sources
- Guidelines: e.g. hypertension guidelines, or management of dyspepsia.
- Visits to other practices / teams, e.g. visiting the local drugs and rehabilitation team.

Grant identified 46 formal and informal methods of needs assessment – see Grant (2002) Learning needs assessment: assessing the need. *BMJ*, **324**, 156–159.

THE PERSONAL DEVELOPMENT PLAN (PDP)

All doctors were expected to have a PDP by April 2000. The PDP should contain the following information:

1. What the planned CPD activity is.
2. Its intended date of completion.
3. How the educational need was identified.

4. The changes to practice that will occur on completion of the CPD.
5. The dates for completion of the changes detailed in (4).

For example, a locum doctor may identify from his PUNs and DENs a knowledge gap regarding the treatment of drug addicts in Primary Care.

1. The planned CPD may be to review the practice's protocol and discuss it with a partner who has an interest in addiction management.
2. It may take 2–3 hours (perhaps a few lunch hours) to read the protocol and an email to the interested partner to clarify matters.
3. The need was identified by an inability to manage the clinical needs of a drug addict in surgery.
4. In future, when working at practices that manage drug addiction, the locum will be able to write out the correct prescriptions and feel more confident about managing addiction.
5. Over the next two months, the locum doctor can keep a list of five addiction patients that he managed and review their records to see if follow-up consultations agreed with his management plans.

He can disseminate the information he has learnt to other locums when they meet at non-principals' groups. The information can be shared, discussed and analysed, thus reinforcing his learning. The doctor may read the clinical governance report that the practice has produced – this should give him information about the effectiveness of his practice.

LEARNING POINTS

- Kaufman's discrepancy model of needs analysis
- SWOT analysis
- Personal reflection
- PUNS and DENS
- 360° feedback
- MAAG

If the examiner wants to push you further, he will ask:

- Name the different ways in which a doctor can identify his learning needs.
- What are the possible advantages and disadvantages of these methods?
- Which method(s) will you choose and why?
- On reviewing your work in six months, how would you know if you had chosen the correct tool for identifying your learning needs?

ADDITIONAL INFORMATION

CPD and clinical governance
CPD was defined in *A first class service* (1998) as:

'a process of life-long learning for all individuals and teams which meets the needs of patients and delivers the health care outcomes and healthcare priorities of the NHS, and which enables professionals to expand to fulfil their potential.'

Therefore doctors need to assess their learning needs, undertake learning that is relevant to those needs, bring their learning back to their practice to improve the quality of patient care. CPD plays a key part in improving quality – it is part of the clinical governance agenda.

Patient satisfaction surveys

A variety of patient satisfaction surveys are available. The client-focused evaluations programme (see: http://latis.ex.ac.uk/_cfep) examines the individual doctors' interpersonal skills.

Significant event auditing (SEA)

Significant event auditing covers positive practice, adverse events and critical incidents. Some significant events are adverse events – when something has clearly gone wrong, such as a prescribing error or administering the incorrect vaccination. The team needs to establish what happened, what was preventable and how to respond.

A critical incident is a half-way house – an event that may indicate sub-standard care, but which might also occur by chance, such as an allergic reaction to a drug or a teenage pregnancy. Critical incidents are theoretically avoidable and possible pointers to deficiencies in care.

SEA needs a blame-free culture – it needs a willingness to honestly acknowledge genuine mistakes, reflect on them and improve practice, so reducing the potential for mistakes in the future.

SEA is not an appropriate technique in cases where legal action is anticipated or where individual incompetence is suspected.

As the aim is to be supportive of colleagues, feedback should be constructive, and should explore possible alternatives for the future. This links it to evidence-based practice, and the adoption of guidelines and best practice.

Significant events are often emotional experiences – unlike audits which are rather dry, SEs are remembered. SEA is effective because it uses emotional engagement to consolidate improvements in patient care.

Westcott R *et al.* (2000) Significant event audit in practice: a preliminary study. *Family practice*, **17**(2), 173–179.

The aim of the study was to identify participants' perceptions of the benefits and problems associated with SEA in the context of primary care, and to derive suggestions which might improve the process of SEA. The study concluded that SEA is a powerful tool, which contributes to teambuilding, enhanced communication, and improvement in patient care. However, its implementation requires sensitive handling for optimal benefit, and to minimise difficulties. The study goes on to describe suggestions to facilitate these processes.

Norman GI, Shannon SI *et al.* (2004) The need for needs assessment in continuing medical education. *BMJ*, **328**(7446), 999–1001.

A fundamental gap remains between the learning needs of the individual practitioner and the priority educational needs identified by bodies for continuing medical education for course offerings. The two are not synonymous.

- Learning needs are personal, specific, and identified by the individual learner through practice experience, reflection, questioning, practice audits, self-assessment tests, peer review, and other sources.
- In contrast, educational needs can be defined as the interests or perceived needs of a whole target audience and can be identified through surveys, focus groups, analysis of regional practice patterns, and evaluations of CME (continuing medical education) programmes. They are necessarily more general than learning needs.

An example of an educational needs assessment is a discrepancy or 'gap' analysis, in which current practice behaviour is compared with an ideal or accepted standard of practice. In contrast, an exploration of the issues that created the gap, in individual cases, would identify the learning needs.

RELEVANT LITERATURE

Pringle M, Bradley C, Carmichael CM *et al.* (1995) **Significant event auditing: a study of the feasibility and potential of case based auditing in primary medical care.** Occasional paper no. 70. *RCGP Publications.*

Secretary of State for Health (1998) **A first class service. Quality in the new NHS.** *NHS Executive,* Leeds. www.nhshistory.net/a_first_class_service.htm

Van Zwanenberg T and Harrison J (editors) (2003) **Clinical governance in primary care.** 2nd edition. *The Radcliffe Medical Press,* Abingdon.

For a good overview and links to the main political documents, see http://www.trentdeanery.nottingham.ac.uk/pri_continuing.htm

Kings College London has a website to help doctors prepare for life-long learning. See http://gppc.kcl.ac.uk/guide/links.htm

There are very few studies evaluating CME. See

Davis DA, Thomson MA, Oxman AD, Haynes RB (1995) **Changing physician performance. A systematic review of the effect of continuing medical education strategies.** *Journal of American Medical Association,* **274,** 700–705.

Haynes RB, Davis DA, McKibben A, Tugwell P (1984) **A critical appraisal of the efficacy of CME.** *JAMA,* **251,** 61–64.

Kaufman R and English FW (1979) **Needs assessment: concept and application.** *Educational Technology Publications,* Englewood Cliffs, NJ.

Stein L (1981) **The effectiveness of continuing medical education – eight research reports.** *Journal of Medical Education,* **56,** 103–110.

This question tests the doctor's personal and professional growth in the context of working with colleagues.

The way in which GP education is delivered has changed. Personal development plans (PDPs) have replaced Postgraduate educational allowance (PGEA).

PDPs promote learner-centredness – the learners

- identify their learning needs,
- develop plans to undertake learning and then
- evaluate their learning.

PDPs move away from a learning programme that is delivered by teachers around their chosen subjects with the learners being passive recipients of the knowledge. PDPs put the learners in charge of their learning. The PDP includes:

- A needs assessment – how the learner identifies his learning needs, using PUNs and DENs, reflection, complaints etc.
- Topics that he intends to study.
- Methods that he will use to complete the study – internet searches, asking colleagues, reading a book or journal, attending a course.
- An evaluation of his learning – how he will know when his needs have been met? The doctor may develop:
  - new skills (e.g. he may now be proficient at injecting joints),
  - new knowledge (e.g. he may feel more confident in future practice) and
  - new attitudes (he may respond differently to demands – e.g. he may feel less anxious with 'heartsink' patients)
- A plan for disseminating and sharing his new knowledge.

Will a journal club (JC) help the doctor to meet the requirements of his PDP?

I think Journal Club is a good idea because:

- It provides a good opportunity to meet with doctors to discuss evidence-based medicine and the latest treatments. Providing the papers are applicable to my practice, it would keep me up to date.
- The work load is shared – someone new presents a topic each week or fortnight.
- Journal club is a fixed commitment – I would be expected to attend and I would set aside time for preparation.
- The group resources are pooled – if I am not good at statistics, someone can help me with this difficult area. I learn more from the group than I would learn on my own.
- I would be able to share my learning with other doctors and the group discussion could generate new ideas for my own practice.
- Journal club provides the opportunity to meet with other local doctors – we provide each other with mutual support and the discussion of EBM may actually be a secondary activity.

Criteria from PDP	Advantages	Disadvantages
Will JC help the doctor to identify his learning needs?	The doctor may identify blindspots. For example, after discussing a paper on atrial fibrillation, he may realize that he does not refer patients for ECHOs appropriately.	The doctor is not identifying his learning needs from his work. These needs are the most relevant and carry the highest priority. Fulfilling them will have the biggest impact on his practice.
Are the papers discussed at JC relevant to the doctor?	A GP-based journal club has the potential to discuss very important and relevant topics for general practice. Discussion of the literature with colleagues is a good way of making EBM applicable to local practice. For example all the doctors may decide to use ACE-I as first line anti-hypertensives in young patients in the future.	The journal club may not cover the doctor's identified learning needs. It may fail to influence his working behaviour through its lack of relevance and generalisability. For example, the GPwSI in dermatology may discuss papers on treatments not commonly prescribed in general practice.
Will the method of study employed at JC be suitable to the doctor?	Journal club provides the opportunity to develop the GP's critical appraisal and presentation skills. It also provides a forum for general discussion.	Not all GPs enjoy learning in a group. The rates of learning and the topics for discussion need to be negotiated by the group. The GP may prefer to work independently and at his own pace.
How will the doctor know whether JC improved his practice?	His critical appraisal, presentation and group work skills improve over time. He may get feedback from the group and he may feel more confident.	Evaluation of changes made to his actual day-to-day practice may be difficult to demonstrate unless he does before and after audits.
Will JC help the doctor to disseminate and share his learning?	The journal club provides a forum for discussion and doctors will share their experiences of implementing EBM – good practice is fostered.	Journal club can create a two-tier system. Some doctors may be discouraged by the academic nature of the method of learning and their non-attendance means that good practice will not be shared.

I think Journal Club is not a good idea because:

- It may not address my identified learning needs. I may be quite good at EBM. My learning needs may be centred around developing a diabetic service and I am unlikely to learn these specific skills at Journal Club.
- Journal club is potentially time-consuming. I would need to prepare for the meeting, travel to the group and discuss ideas for an hour or two. I may be able to learn EBM that is directly applicable to me by conducting my own on-line searches based on my PUNs and DENs.
- It may take up an entire afternoon or evening and it may not suit my home situation. The programme may not be flexible enough to suit and I would prefer to do internet-based study such as on-line *BMJ*-learning from my desk top at work or at home.
- I already attend weekly practice meetings, local PCT meetings and meet with the Young Principals Group – I do not need to attend Journal Club to meet my social and support needs.
- I am a self-motivated individual learner, who likes to solve real patient-based problems. My learning style is therefore not compatible with the reflective learning style required of a journal club. I may not enjoy group interaction.

If you choose not to attend Journal Club, how else can you address your learning needs? I can undertake:

- Individual learning:
  - Reading journals (such as the *BMJ* or *Clinical Evidence*),
  - Undertaking internet searches (such as prodigy, www.clinicalevidence.nhs.uk or Bandolier)
  - Attending appropriate study days (such as the Appraisers course)
- Group learning:
  - Practice meetings, including audit and significant event audit meetings
  - Update meetings where the practices meet on a regular basis and invite local consultants to discuss the local service provision
  - Special interest meetings, such as women's health or dermatology updates
  - Balint groups or Higher Professional Education group meetings
- Attending courses or undertaking work placements:
  - For example, attending a minor surgery workshop or doing supervised sessions in a family planning clinic for the Diploma of Family Planning

LEARNING POINTS

- Personal development plans (PDPs) have replaced Postgraduate educational allowance (PGEA)
- PDPs contain a needs assessment of learning, identified study methods or opportunities and an evaluation of learning
- Learning styles (Honey and Mumford)
- The primary gain of journal club may be skills in EBM, the secondary gain may be the social support from local doctors

ADDITIONAL INFORMATION

Learning styles

Honey and Mumford (1989) describe learners as activists, reflectors, theorists or pragmatists based on their preferred learning style. They argue that if attention is paid to learning styles, then more effective learning can take place.

Kolb (1984) describes a model of learning called experiential learning – the learner begins with an experience ('concrete experience') which is followed by reflection ('reflective observation'). The reflection is then assimilated into a theory ('abstract conceptualisation'). The theory is tested in new situations ('active experimentation') which in turn gives rise to new concrete experiences. A recurring cycle of learning occurs.

Honey and Mumford built on Kolb's work by connecting a learning style to each stage of the learning cycle (as shown in *Figure 1*). Depending on the preferred learning style, the learner will enter into the learning cycle at any of the four points.

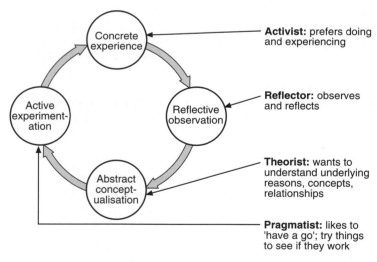

Figure 1. Typology of learners cycle. Reproduced from *http://www.learningand teaching.info/learning/experience.htm* with permission.

RELEVANT LITERATURE

Honey P and Mumford A (1986) **The learning styles questionnaire.** *Peter Honey Publications Limited*, Maidenhead, Berks.

Howard J (2001) **Small groups in Mersey Region 1989–98. A survey of activity in general practice.** *Education for General Practice*. Vol. 12. No. 1, pp. 47–56.

Knowles MS (1984) **Androgogy in action: applying modern principles of adult learning.** Jossey Bass, San Francisco.

Kolb D (1984) **Experiental learning: experience as a source of learning and development.** Prentice Hall, Englewoods Cliff, NJ.

Rugani A (2000) **The GP's guide to personal development plans.** *Radcliffe Medical Press*, Oxford.

Schon DA (1983) **The reflective practitioner. How professionals think in action.** *Basic Books Inc.*, USA.

This question tests the doctor's personal and professional growth in the context of caring for patients and/or working with colleagues.

Appraisal is a formative tool in which a doctor's discussion of his educational and professional developmental needs is facilitated by a peer. By formative we mean that the outcome measured is the growth or improvement of the doctor, whereas by summative (as in summative assessment), we mean that the outcome is a pass or fail. Appraisal is not a test; it does not have pass/fail outcomes – it is not an assessment of a doctor's performance.

The appraisal discussion needs to occur annually. The appraisee is responsible for collating a personal development plan (PDP), and reflecting on his future plans. The appraiser is responsible for organising the venue, reviewing the PDP folder at least two weeks before the interview and facilitating the discussion. Both parties complete the Department of Health forms (form 5 and PDP template). See www.doh.gov.uk/gpappraisal.

THERE ARE FIVE FORMS:

Form 1: Basic details – such as practice address and qualifications.

Form 2: Current medical activities – such as a description of the doctor's daily activities and clinical work.

Form 3: Material for appraisal. This forms the bulk of the appraisal. The doctor is asked to comment on how his work has improved since his last appraisal, his views on his continuing development needs and an overview of the drivers and obstacles to his plans for change. The doctor needs to provide documents in support of this, so preparation for appraisal involves collecting this data. The documents list includes:

- Personal reflection: sticky moments; PUNs and DENs (clinical diary)
- Reflective reading and internet searches
- Summaries of learning points from meetings attended, or a list of PGEA events attended
- Referral rates
- Feedback from patients, complaints and peers (patient satisfaction surveys, practice appraisal documentation, 360° feedback)
- Audit, significant event audit and MAAG data
- PACT data
- The doctor's personal development plan
- The practice deed
- Appraisal documentation from outside jobs (for example, in GPs with special interests or doctors who work for the PCT / deanery)
- Research grant applications and publications

Form 4: Summary of appraisal discussion with an agreed action plan and a personal development plan. This form is completed by appraiser and appraisee following their discussion.

Form 5: Detailed confidential account of appraisal interview. This is an optional form for the appraisee to complete, to note down his reflections and plans arising from the appraisal process.

Personal preparation (Lewin's model of change, Iles and Sutherland, 2001):

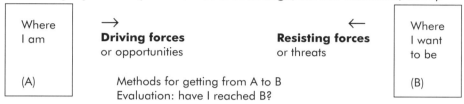

STEP-WISE PREPARATION

- The doctor can get direction from *Good medical practice for general practitioners*. This describes the criteria for an 'excellent' GP.
- Using standards from *Good medical practice for general practitioners*, the doctor writes down his goals ('where he wants to be').
- By reviewing his current practice, he identifies 'where he is'. He completes a needs assessment (see chapter on 'keeping up to date').
- He identifies the gaps between where he is and where he wants to be, and prioritises his learning needs. The prioritisation takes into account the needs of the practice (from the Practice Development Plan), the patients and the PCT (who may be offering incentives for change).
- The doctor identifies the tools or methods for addressing these needs. This includes self-directed learning; attending study days (e.g. how to set up a diabetic clinic); meeting with other professionals (study groups / Balint groups).
- The doctor evaluates whether he achieved his goals and provides evidence to this effect. This may include personal reflection, changes made to practice protocols, evidence from re-auditing, and a second round of patient and peer surveys.

ADDITIONAL INFORMATION

1. Cross M and White P (2004) Personal development plans: the *Wessex experience. Education for Primary Care*, **15**(2), 205–12.

GPs in Wessex were asked by questionnaire to express their opinions on aspects of professional development, PDPs and their implementation. A space was also provided for free text comments on any aspect of the questionnaire.

- An 81% response rate was achieved, with 277 completed questionnaires.
- Of these, 64% of respondents claimed to have submitted their PDP primarily to gain PGEA accreditation.
- The majority believed that professional development helps keep GPs up to date.
- Over 50% of GPs regard the completion of a PDP as a 'hoop-jumping' exercise.
- Educational tools were valued as aids to learning, with 81% regarding significant event auditing (SEA) as favourable.
- Educational tools such as SEAs, Patients' Unmet Needs (PUNs) and Doctors' Educational Needs (DENs) were highly regarded.

2. Cross M and White P (2004) Practice professional development plans: the Wessex experience. *Education for Primary Care*, **15**(2), 213–19.

Some practices regarded the implementation of a practice plan as a teambuilding exercise.

- Educational tools such as significant event auditing (SEA) and reflecting on practice were by consensus beneficial.

- 75% of respondents felt that sufficient protected time was not available, and that professional development work should take place within practice hours.
- The role of the practice manager was regarded as pivotal in taking practice plans forward and creating a teambuilding effect.
- Facilitation was regarded as useful, with lack of feedback contributing to a negative effect on completing a practice plan.

3. St George IM, Kaigas T *et al*. (2004) Assessing the competence of practising physicians in New Zealand, Canada, and the United Kingdom: progress and problems. *Family Medicine*, **36**(3), 172–7.

Members of the public expect practising physicians to be competent. They expect poorly performing physicians to be identified and either helped or removed from practice. 'Maintenance of professional standards' by continuing education (i.e. annual appraisal) does not identify the poorly performing doctor; *assessment* of clinical performance is necessary for that. A single, valid, reliable, and practical screening tool has yet to be devised to identify physicians whose practice is suboptimal.

4. St George IM (2004) Assessing performance 2: how should the underperforming doctor be identified? *New Zealand Family Physician*, **31**(2), 112–14.
   http://www.rnzcgp.org.nz/NZFP/Issues/April2004/StGeorge_Apr04.pdf

This article applies Wilson's screening criteria to the whole population of doctors to identify the poor performers. It says that the NHS has adopted a three-pronged approach to identify poor performers:

1. periodic screening: revalidation which incorporates annual appraisal. (Appraisal is formative – helping the doctor develop. Revalidation is summative – the doctor's licence to continue practising is either granted or not. Therefore revalidation is a pass/fail test, i.e. an assessment of the doctor's performance.)
2. responsive reviews on receipt of concerns: the GMC has a responsive system of competence reviews
3. employer credentialling activities: the National Clinical Assessment Authority (NCAA) reviews the doctor's competence on receipt of complaints.

5. Van Zwanenberg T (2004) Revalidation: the purpose needs to be clear. *BMJ*, **328**(7441), 684–6.

From 1 January 2005 every UK doctor will need a licence to practise. Most doctors will be able to secure revalidation of their licence by annual appraisal and by showing that they are compliant with local clinical governance requirements and free of any serious unresolved concerns about their fitness to practice.

6. Bruce D, Phillips K *et al*. (2004) Revalidation for general practitioners: randomised comparison of two revalidation models. *BMJ*, **328**(7441), 687–91.

The aim of the RCT was to compare two models of revalidation for general practitioners. 66 Scottish general practitioners (principals and non-principals) participated, 53 of whom completed the revalidation folders. Two revalidation models were compared:

- a minimum criterion based model with revalidation as the primary purpose, and
- an educational outcome model with emphasis on combining revalidation with continuing professional development.

Results:

- The criterion model was preferred by general practitioners.
- Summative assessment of the folders showed reasonable inter-rater reliability.

Conclusions: The criterion model provides a practical and acceptable model for general practitioners to use when preparing for revalidation.

7. In August 2004, the RCGP issued a consultation document – *Portfolio of evidence of professional standards for GPs* – and asked for comments from members, other Royal Colleges and medical institutions. The RCGP will produce a revalidation toolkit mapped to the criteria, standards and evidence in this document. It will help all types of GPs to gather evidence for their portfolios and enable them to demonstrate their professional standards. See: http://www.rcgp.org.uk/press/docs/revalidation.pdf

8. The National Association of Primary Care Educators (NAPCE) has compiled an *ABC of GP appraisal* documents. There are thirteen documents in all. Titles are: Definitions and aims of appraisal; Quality assurance in practice; Selection of appraisers; Training of appraisers; Keeping appraisers up to date; Organisation of appraisal; The appraisal interview; Appraisal: the paperwork; The problem appraisal; Evaluation of the GP appraisal process; Using the results of GP appraisal; How to write an annual appraisal report; and GP appraisal: the PCO's responsibility.
See: http://www.natpact.nhs.uk/cms/380.php#docs

WHAT GPs COULD BE ASKED AT THEIR APPRAISAL (from the NHS appraisal toolkit)

Section one – current job

- Main responsibilities
- Strengths
- Aspects of the job that give the greatest satisfaction
- Problems and how they could be solved
- Major changes to your job over the last year, positive and negative
- Concerns about changes
- Changes needed to enable you to work more effectively and/or with greater satisfaction
- Activities or achievements

Section two – clinical performance
- Examples of clinical governance
- Significant events in the practice and in your own work
- Feedback from patients
- Relationships with patients and ways they could be improved
- Relationships with team
- Details of continuing medical education and how it fits with practice priorities
- How well have you met last year's goals? Any difficulties and how they could be overcome
- Concerns about probity and how to deal with them
- Is your health affecting your work or vice versa?

Section three – involvement in practice development and relationships to practice / PCT and NHS priorities
- Developments that have prompted teamwork
- Other contributions to developing services in practice
- How effective is your practice in delivering service outcomes?
- What resources would help you and your practice become more effective?

Section four – career interests
- Career interests within the practice and any other areas of work
- What would help you achieve this?
- How do you see your career developing?

Section five – wider interest
- Role in NHS management, IT, PCT, health improvement task groups
- Teaching and training commitments
- Willingness to extend involvement in any other areas
- Could you offer any learning opportunities to colleagues across the PCT?

RELEVANT LITERATURE

GMC (2001) **Good medical practice**. Third edition. London. http://www.gmc-uk.org/standards/good.htm

Iles, V and Sutherland K (2001) **Organisational change: managing change in the NHS** [online]. *NHS SDO R and D Programme*, London. Available from www.sdo.lshtm.ac.uk

This RCGP resource contains guidance, toolkits and forms which help GPs (including non-principals and trainees) complete the appraisal and revalidation process. http://www.rcgp.org.uk/webmaster/gpportalframes/index.asp

NHS appraisal toolkit: https://www.appraisals.nhs.uk/

Appraisal for GPs with specialist interests: http://www.gpiag.org/education/gpwsi_discussion.php

Appraisal for non-principals: http://www.nasgp.org.uk/cpd/appraisal/index.htm

For revalidation information, see http://www.gmc-uk.org/revalidation/information_and_papers/l_and_r_formal_guidance_for_docs.pdf

This question tests the doctor's personal and professional growth in the context of caring for patients and working with colleagues.

Audit is an important clinical governance (CG) activity. The aim of CG is to explicitly demonstrate that good quality care is being delivered and that continual improvements in care are being made. Clinical audit aims to lead to an improvement in the quality of health service so that:

- patient care is improved
- the professionalism of staff is enhanced
- resources are used efficiently
- continuing education is focused
- administration is efficient
- accountability is demonstrated.

Under the new GMS contract, doctors are remunerated for providing evidence of good quality care. The evidence usually derives from practice audits. For example, there are 121 Quality and Outcomes points available for secondary prevention in CHD. To attain these points, audit activity must occur in the practice.

The above question can be answered in one of two ways:

- Using a managing change model: plan, study, do, act (PDSA cycle)
- Using a mentoring model: Driscoll's (2000) **'What?'** model of facilitating change.

The framework of Driscoll's **'What?'** model comprises:

- **'What?'**: A description of the events. What happened?
- **'So what?'**: An analysis of the event. What resulted from these events? How did people feel?
- **'Now what?'**: Proposed actions following the event. What can you do now and should this occur again, what could you do differently?

WHAT?

The doctor could explore how Dr A feels about audit and the reasons for his reluctance:

- Computer illiterate – unable to construct searches. He is keen but lacking in the necessary skills.
- About to retire – not keen to learn new tricks!
- Fails to see the value of audit – he has never had a patient complaint, so why should he change?
- Political ideology: he resists being ordered about by the PCT and sees no reason for demonstrating accountability – people should simply trust him.

- Practice politics – audit is an activity of younger doctors; he would prefer to manage other aspects of the practice.

The doctor could ask him questions that challenge Dr A's assumptions:

- What does he intend to do for his appraisal and revalidation?
- Does he think that not being able to audit is perceived as a problem by the practice?
- What does he perceive the obstacles in undertaking an audit to be? How could these obstacles be tackled?
- What are the possible benefits of auditing?
- If he were to undertake audit, what educational or support mechanisms would he like to have in place?

The purpose of asking open questions is to come to a shared understanding of the problem and possible solutions. The aim is not to tell Dr A what to do and how to do it, but rather to facilitate a change. Dr A must come to an understanding of his learning needs and how best to address them. Dr A may dislike attending a computer workshop update and may prefer one-to-one informal tuition with the audit clerk.

SO WHAT?

What does Dr A perceive to be the worst case scenario and is this likely to happen? Does he fear failure? Is he willing to risk the antagonism of the rest of the partnership for fear of losing face?

Should he decide not to participate in audit, what would he prefer to do? How would the rest of the practice feel about this?

NOW WHAT?

What arrangements can be made to help him change? Practical steps need to be discussed. Which audits is he most interested in doing?

After this discussion, the doctor could ask Dr A to summarise his vision – what would he like to achieve in the next six months; what would aid him; and how does he intend to tackle any obstacles?

Dr A asks you to explain the basic principles of audit. What would you say?

Ideas
Based on Dr A's interests, I would discuss possible ideas for audit and allow him to choose an example, such as 'Patients on thyroxine should have their TSH checked every 15 months.'

Justification for the audit
He would need to justify why he is checking the TSH every 15 months – is this recommendation based on good research or local protocols? He needs to quote

the source of the recommendation. In some cases, he may need to search the literature and appraise the evidence.

Criteria chosen

Criteria should be SMART (specific, measurable, achievable, reliable, timely) measures of quality.

With regard to thyroxine:

- Specific: was the TSH checked – yes or no?
- Measurable: the number of patients who had their TSH checked can be counted.
- Achievable: the audit is not beyond the scope of general practice and is suitable for a beginner. There are a limited number of READ codes in the search, unlike LFTs and statins where multiple READ codes for the different statins are needed.
- Reliable: the search is measuring what you actually want it to measure and you can use this result to improve patient care. For example, you want to identify patients who have not had their TSH measured so that you can offer them a test.
- Timely: the practice has a limited number of patients on thyroxine so the audit should be quick and easy to do even with manual note checks.

Standards set

Standards are the levels of care you are prepared to accept. The new GMS contract awards six points if 90% of patients on thyroxine have had their TSH measured in the last 15 months. After discussion with the PHCT, you may wish to set a higher percentage or stricter time frame to allow a safety margin.

Data collection

Discuss with the audit lead how best to 'catch' all patients on thyroxine. Which READ codes are needed? Does everybody READ code appropriately and how would you identify patients whose diagnosis and results were free-texted?

Results and changes

Discuss the results of the initial data collection. Present the results to the PHCT in a simple format. Agree changes and identify persons responsible for implementing the changes.

Second data collection

After implementing the change, the practice needs to reaudit. Have the changes resulted in the standards being met? If not, further action needs to be taken with a planned review date, i.e. go around the audit cycle again.

Conclusions

Is the practice delivering high quality care to hypothyroid patients? What evidence is there to support this?

LEARNING POINTS

- PDSA model of managing change
- Driscoll's model of facilitating reflective development
- SMART criteria
- The stages of the audit cycle – completing the loop

If the examiner wants to push you further, he will ask:

- Does audit improve the quality of care delivered by general practice?
- Are there other systems in place to improve the quality of care in general practice?
- What are the possible advantages and disadvantages of audit activity?
- In six months, how will you know if the time spent on audit activity has actually improved the quality of care to your patients?

ADDITIONAL INFORMATION

Lyratzopoulos G and Allen D (2004) How to manage your research and audit work. *BMJ Career Focus*, **328**(7449), 196–197.

Project management is a useful strategy to manage the time and resources needed to produce a good audit. The article describes the seven stages of project management:

1. Define the objective of your audit precisely: one way to focus the audit is by using a SMART format to identify the specific, measured, agreed, realistic, and timed objectives of your audit.
2. Recruit and build a team.
3. Communicate the goals of your audit.
4. Plan carefully.
5. Commit the plan to paper.
6. Check progress. Gantt charts are a useful way of representing and checking that all the tasks are being completed in the correct order and within the required timescale. Software packages such as Microsoft Project can help, but you can do a Gantt chart in Microsoft Excel, which is more widely available.
7. Identify critical success and failure factors. You cannot make carrot soup without carrots. Similarly, critical success factors for your audit might include access to good library facilities, web access, the assistance of someone who understands READ codes and search principles, and the availability of a word processor.

RELEVANT LITERATURE

The Bath VTS website provides an excellent step by step 'how to do an audit' for those who have little or no experience of clinical audit in a general practice setting. See http://www.mharris.eurobell.co.uk/contents.htm

Clinical Governance Support Team: www.modern.nhs.uk/scripts/default.asp?site_id=18

For an example of a Gantt chart, see www.mindtools.com/pages/article/newPPM_03.htmNational Institute for Clinical Excellence: www.nice.org.uk/

National Primary Care Development Team: www.npdt.org

For information on project management, see http://www.phel.gov.uk/healthknowledge/svrSearchHK.asp and www.mphe.man.ac.uk.

For further information on SMART, see www.projectsmart.co.uk/smart_goals.html.

For advice on team-building see http://ollie.dcccd.edu/mgmt1374/book_contents/4directing/teambldg/teambldg.htm

Significant event audits (SEA):

A 46 year old man attends for his annual occupational medical. Asymptomatic microscopic haematuria is found on dipstix. The patient reassures the doctor that he has had haematuria ever since his vasectomy. On closer inspection of his notes, the doctor notices that this is the fourth consecutive year on which haematuria was found. He investigates the patient and an ultrasound picks up a mass suggestive of renal cancer. How can the practice learn from this?

This question tests the doctor's personal and professional growth in the context of caring for patients.

The practice can learn from this critical incident by undertaking a significant event audit (SEA). SEA is defined as a systematic investigation of an individual's case records to improve the care for others. It involves reporting, analysing and learning from adverse events, critical incidents and examples of positive practice.

- Adverse events are instances where something has clearly gone wrong.
- Critical incidents are events where the patient was put at risk but did not actually come to harm – near misses.

In the above case, the doctor involved can complete a significant event form. This is usually available in an electronic or paper format. The completed form containing a brief, anonymised summary should be passed to the chair for discussion at the next SEA meeting. These meetings should be held regularly. The chair structures the discussion and encourages contributions from all participants. The aim is to be supportive and constructive. The chair compiles a written summary of the general conclusions with any actions to be taken, for review at a future specified date.

Significant events include:

- delayed diagnoses
- patient complaints
- new cancer diagnoses
- new cases of stroke or MIs
- prescribing and dispensing errors

The important features of SEA are:

- The practice should have a mechanism for reporting SE. This mechanism should be easily accessible to all staff.
- A blame-free culture should be developed (emulating the airline industry).
- Meetings should be held regularly.
- Everybody should participate, including non-clinical staff.
- Examples of good and less good care should be discussed.
- The care should be analysed and the lessons learnt should be disseminated to the wider PHCT.

- At subsequent meetings, the practice should check that the outcomes of previous meetings are being implemented.

Possible SEA outcomes are that:

- good practice is identified and disseminated.
- the team identifies a learning need and undertakes further research – practise DENs!
- a change in practice is implemented. Local guidelines and protocols may be reviewed and updated based on new evidence.
- it may be that an unfortunate error has occurred from which no new lessons can be learnt, e.g. a traffic jam delays attendance to an emergency home visit.

LEARNING POINTS

- Adverse versus critical incidents
- Mechanism for reporting – SEA
- Blame-free culture – constructive feedback
- Practise DENs

If the examiner wants to push you further, he will ask:
- What makes doctors change their consulting behaviour and improve their clinical skills?
- What are the possible advantages and disadvantages of SEAs?
- Will you share your learning from SEAs with other practices? Will you publish anonymised SEAs on the PCT website?
- What are the possible advantages and disadvantages of disseminating the learning publicly in this way?

ADDITIONAL INFORMATION

McKay J, Bowie P *et al.* (2004) Attitudes to the identification and reporting of significant events in general practice. *Clinical Governance an International Journal*, **9**(2), 96–100.

The new National Patient Safety Agency (NPSA) aims to facilitate the mandatory reporting of relevant significant events. A questionnaire survey of 617 general practitioners was undertaken and 466 responses were received (76 %).

- A minority (18%) agreed the reporting of adverse incidents should be mandatory.
- A majority (73%) agreed that they would be selective in their reporting in a mandatory system.
- Most (75%) favoured a local anonymised system of reporting.
- A difficulty in determining when an event is 'significant' was acknowledged by 41% of respondents.

- 30% agreed significant events were often not acted on.
- Less experienced respondents were more likely to have difficulty in determining when an event is significant (p = 0.01).

The success of the NPSA system may be obstructed by the mandatory requirement to participate and in the difficulty for some in determining when an event is 'significant'.

Dean P, Farooqi A *et al.* (2004) Quality improvement in general practice: the perspective of the primary healthcare team. *Quality in Primary Care*, **12**(3), 201–7.

Members of 17 primary healthcare teams were interviewed regarding the new quality and outcomes framework in general practice. Staff were anxious that quality improvement may be a waste of effort and resources. All team members, especially GPs, were concerned about time and resources. General practitioners and administrative staff expressed concern about the understanding and implementation of the quality process, whereas nurses and members of professions allied to medicine expressed more concerns about teamwork.

RELEVANT LITERATURE

An organisation with a memory (DoH, 2000).
Building a safer NHS for patients (DoH, 2001).
Pringle M, Bradley C, Carmichael C, Wallis H, Moore A (1995) **Significant event auditing.** Occasional paper 70. *Royal College of General Practitioners*, London.
Richie J and Davies S (1995) **Professional negligence: a duty of candid disclosure?** BMJ, **310,** 888–889.
Robinson L, Stacy R, Spencer J, Bhopal R (1995) **Use of facilitated case discussions for significant event auditing.** BMJ, **311,** 315–318.

A patient with Raynaud's phenomenon brings you an article that he has downloaded from the internet. The article describes a study of 14 people with Raynaud's who were successfully treated with acupuncture. He asks for your opinion on the study.

This question tests the doctor's communication skills in the context of caring for patients. It also tests his ability to appraise evidence and discuss research findings with patients in lay terms. Doctors are increasingly asked to interpret information from a variety of sources and are no longer the sole guardians of medical knowledge.

In '*The new consultation: developing doctor–patient communication*', Pendleton *et al.* (2003) advise doctors to improve their communication by:

1. understanding the reasons for the patient's attendance
2. understanding the patient's perspective of the problem
3. sharing that understanding to arrive at an appropriate management plan
4. sharing decisions and responsibility
5. maintaining the doctor–patient relationship
6. considering ongoing problems
7. using time effectively

These are known as the seven tasks of consultation.

The patient may want alternative treatment of his Raynaud's for a variety of reasons:

- He may not have received a good explanation of the condition initially.
- He may be experiencing unacceptable side effects from the medication he is currently receiving.
- His ideas about his illness and his treatment may differ from the medical model. The doctor needs to incorporate the patient's health beliefs into the management plan.

It is important to respect the patient's views even if these differ from the practitioner's. The doctor may offer to research the use of acupuncture in the treatment of Raynaud's in more depth, to offer an evidence-based opinion. An evidence-based approach requires the doctor to:

- Define the research question: 'What are the benefits and harms of acupuncture in the treatment of Raynaud's in an adult patient?'
- Search for the evidence: Consult *Clinical evidence*, although paper references rapidly become outdated. Cochrane, Cinahl and Bandolier are good electronic databases. If systematic reviews are not available, the doctor could then look for well-conducted randomised controlled trials in Medline and the *BMJ*. A medical librarian can undertake much of the research since searches, unless well-defined, can take longer than expected.
- Appraise the evidence for its validity and relevance: Validity may be a

difficult concept for the patient to understand – he may purely focus on the results. A doctor needs to appraise the evidence before accepting the results. He may have to explain to the patient that the construct of the trial was flawed, thus making the results invalid. For example, a trial involving 14 patients may not have sufficient power for the results to be valid. Turning scientific jargon into understandable English may stretch even the best communicators, particularly in a time-limited consultation!

- Seek and incorporate the user's values and preferences – from his research, the doctor may feel that there is insufficient evidence for the use of acupuncture; however, the patient may disagree. The doctor may be trying to act in the patient's best interests by providing evidence-based treatment, but he may be accused of medical paternalism and of not respecting the patient's autonomy.
- Evaluate the effectiveness through planned review against agreed success criteria – in the end, the patient may decide to use acupuncture as a private treatment. A reasonably successful outcome may be the absence of harm and a continuation of the doctor–patient therapeutic alliance. After all, the best treatment is the one the patient will use.

LEARNING POINTS

- Pendleton's seven tasks (2003)
- Databases: Cochrane, Cinahl and Bandolier, Medline
- The doctor–patient therapeutic alliance
- The five tasks of EBM (see chapter on EBM)

If the examiner wants to push you further, he will ask you:

- To name some sources of medical information for patients.
- What are the possible advantages and disadvantages of these different sources of information?
- Is it reasonable to expect doctors to develop their skills of communication and advocacy in the sphere of alternative and complementary medicine?

ADDITIONAL INFORMATION

Wathen B and Dean T (2004) An evaluation of the impact of NICE guidance on GP prescribing. *British Journal of General Practice*, **54**(499), 103–107.

One of the aims of the National Institute for Clinical Excellence (NICE) is to promote faster access to the best treatments. This qualitative study aimed to explore the attitudes of GPs to NICE guidance and to investigate any changes in prescribing patterns. A postal questionnaire, developed from semi-structured interviews, was sent to all GPs within a North Devon PCT to explore factors that were encouraging or discouraging adherence to NICE guidance. There was an 83% response rate.

This study concluded that:

- NICE guidance in isolation had little impact on GP prescribing.
- where the guidance coincided with information from other sources, or personal experience, there was some evidence that technology appraisals triggered an increase in prescribing, but that this was not always sustained.
- the recommendations of NICE concerning zanamivir were universally rejected and there was evidence that this had undermined confidence in NICE recommendations in general.

Coomaramasamy A and Khan KS (2004) What is the evidence that postgraduate teaching in evidence-based medicine changes anything?: a systematic review. *BMJ*, **329**(7473), 1017–19.

The aim of this systematic review was to address the question: is classroom-based teaching or clinically integrated teaching of EBM more effective at improving the knowledge, skills, attitudes and behaviour of graduates?

The review concluded that:

- stand-alone teaching improved knowledge but not skills, attitudes, or behaviour.
- clinically integrated teaching improved knowledge, skills, attitudes, and behaviour.
- teaching of evidence-based medicine should be moved from classrooms to clinical practice to achieve improvements in substantial outcomes.

This question tests the doctor's communication skills in the context of caring for patients. In answering this question, two approaches spring to mind.

- The question can be considered in terms of a consultation model which is useful for navigating challenging patient–doctor dynamics, or
- In ethical terms, the pros and cons of each action may be considered before deciding on a morally justifiable course of action.

Pendleton's Model (2003) advises doctors:

- **To understand the reasons for the patient's attendance.**
  The father may be concerned in view of the patient's past history – is this an example of learned health-seeking behaviour?
  The family may be travelling on holiday and the father may want the problem resolved quickly before a long car journey or flight.
  The father may believe that antibiotics shorten the duration of ear infections and reduce pain – his health beliefs.
  The doctor performs an appropriate physical examination and shares his findings with the patient – is this impacted wax, otitis externa, otitis media or a foreign body?

- **Taking into account the patient's perspective, to achieve a shared understanding about the problem and about the evidence and options for management.**
  Establish the patient's agenda. Doctors are guilty of making assumptions. Does the patient want symptom relief or is the father asking your opinion on his fitness to attend school or go on holiday? Does the patient have an immunodeficiency, such as HIV or an IgA deficiency, that places him at greater risk?
  Discuss his reasons for believing that antibiotics are effective – gently challenge his health beliefs.
  Discuss the evidence-based treatment of acute otitis media in simple, jargon-free terms.
  del Mar *et al.* (1997) showed that antibiotics only benefit 14% of children who are still in pain 24 hours after presentation. However, antibiotics double the risk of vomiting, diarrhoea and rashes.
  After sharing your examination findings and discussing the research evidence with the father, check to see if his health beliefs have altered. The father may have appreciated the time you took in assessing his child's problem and is less likely to feel 'fobbed off' with advice on analgesia. In this way you have achieved concordance (see chapter on patient-centred consulting).

- **To enable the patient to choose an appropriate action for each problem.**
  - Consider options and implications
  - Choose the most appropriate course of action

Options:

1. Give antibiotics: Antibiotics may be indicated. However, there is evidence to suggest that antibiotic prescribing in acute earache is unnecessary. GPs can be influenced into giving antibiotics by several factors. These include pressure from the patient, time pressures within the consultation, precedent set by other doctors or themselves in previous consultations, and pressure from the pharmaceutical industry. However, prescribing in this situation may serve to medicalise the condition and encourage re-attendance for future episodes. It also has implications for promoting antibiotic resistance.

2. Withhold antibiotics and re-attend if worsens: The patient may not understand the difference between viral and bacterial ear infections. The patient may see the doctor as being in a position of power and may resent the over-riding of his wishes.

3. Provide simple analgesics and/or a patient information leaflet: Non-steroidal anti-inflammatories are superior to placebo in the treatment of earache. McFarlane *et al.* (1997) found that patient information leaflets are effective at reducing reconsultation rates and increasing patient satisfaction.

4. Provide a delayed script: The strategy of the patient collecting the script for antibiotics if their symptoms have not improved in 48 hours is effective (Little *et al.*, 1997).

My course of action: My message to the father would be that most children with acute otitis media do not suffer adverse sequelae without antibiotics. The number needed to treat (NNT) for 1 child to benefit (resolution of symptoms 1 day sooner on average) from initial antibiotic therapy is between 7 and 20 (http://www.emedicine.com/emerg/topic393.htm). Try to negotiate a management plan that is mutually acceptable. Provide the patient with options. When the patient chooses an option, he is more likely to commit to the treatment plan.

- **To enable the patient to manage the problem.**
  - Discuss the patient's ability to take appropriate actions
  - Agree doctor and patient actions and responsibilities

  The patient can re-attend or he can collect a script if the problem worsens over 48 hours. The doctor will be responsible for reassessing the problem or providing advice if complications occur (safety netting).

- **To consider other problems.**
  - Not yet presented
  - Continuing problems
  - At-risk factors

  This may not be applicable to all consultations. However, if the patient has experienced many infections and has been poorly for some time, it is worth considering whether there is an underlying reason for the ill health, such as an immunodeficiency or even a social problem.

- **To use time appropriately.**
  - In the consultation
  - In the longer term

Spending a great deal of time with one patient over a self-limiting minor illness, especially in the middle of a busy surgery, may cause you to run late and consultations with less assertive, sicker patients may be compromised. On the other hand, a long consultation in which you strive to achieve concordance may improve the doctor–patient relationship and reduce the frequency of consulting. Patients are more satisfied with longer consultations.

- **To establish and maintain a relationship with the patient which helps to achieve the other tasks.**
  A once-off unnecessary prescription for antibiotics may be the price to pay for maintaining a harmonious doctor–patient relationship. However, such prescribing behaviour may reinforce the patient's health beliefs regarding antibiotics and further promote dependence on unnecessary prescribing.

An ethical model can also be applied.

Autonomy – The father has responsibility for his child's health. However, to make an informed decision, he needs to be aware of the risks and benefits of antibiotics and needs to be informed about alternative treatments.

Beneficence – By advising on current best practice, you are treating in the patient's best interests.

Non-maleficence – By excluding serious pathology and by making follow-up arrangements should the condition worsen (safety netting), you are reducing potential harm to your patient. By giving antibiotics for a self-limiting condition, you are potentially exposing the patient to serious side effects such as anaphylaxis and more minor ones such as rashes.

Justice – Doctors must try to distribute limited resources (time, money, and expensive treatments) fairly. On average a GP would expect to see 100 cases of otitis media a year, amounting to 1.5 million episodes in England and Wales each year.

LEARNING POINTS

- Pendleton's consultation model
- NNT with antibiotics in OM is 7–20
- Concordance
- The average GP sees 100 cases of OM each year

If the examiner wants to push you further, he will ask:

- What are the possible advantages and disadvantages of each of the options?
- Which option will you choose and why?
- On auditing your work in six months, how would you know if you had chosen the correct option?

ADDITIONAL INFORMATION

Lipman T (2004) The doctor, his patient, and the computerized evidence-based guideline. *Journal of Evaluation in Clinical Practice*, **10**(2), 163–76.

The reductionist assumptions underlying the construction of evidence-based guidelines from systematic reviews lead to inflexible recommendations on the management of disease. Anthropologists and sociologists make an important distinction between scientifically defined diseases and the culturally constructed experience of illness. Because GPs deal with patients suffering illness that may or may not result from disease, disease-centred guidelines often conflict with their needs and wishes. The development of evidence-based medicine (EBM) was intended as a tool to help doctors make sense of evidence in the context of individual patients' problems. Few GPs are skilled in it, and it has been appropriated by powerful expert groups such as guidelines developers and the pharmaceutical industry. It is suggested that more understanding of EBM by GPs leads to better-informed decision-making by them and their patients.

RELEVANT LITERATURE

Del Mar C, Glasziou P, Hayem M (1997) **Are antibiotics indicated as initial treatment for children with acute otitis media? A meta-analysis.** *BMJ*, **314**: 1526–9.

Little P, Gould C, Williamson I (1997). **Reattendance and complications in a randomised trial of prescribing strategies for sore throat; the medicalising effect of prescribing antibiotics.** *British Medical Journal* **315**: 350–352.

Mcfarlane JT, Holmes WF and McFarlane RM (1997). **Reducing reconsultations for acute lower respiratory tract illness with an information leaflet; a randomised controlled study of patients in primary care.** *British Journal of General Practice* **47**: 719–722.

Rollnick S, Seale C, Rees M, Butler C, Kinnersley P and Anderson L (2001) **Inside the routine general practice consultation: an observational study of consultations for sore throats.** *Family Practice.***18(5):** 506–510. http://fampra.oupjournals.org/cgi/content/full/18/5/506

Acute otitis media: http://www.clinicalevidence.com/ceweb/conditions/chd/0301/0301.jsp

American website on evidence based medicine: http://www.emedicine.com/emerg/topic393.htm

Your partner is keen to offer homeopathy during working hours in your practice. How would you respond?

This question tests the doctor's communication skills, professional growth and work with colleagues.

The question raises several issues:

- The partnership agreement
- The evidence for complementary and alternative medicines (CAM)
- Ethical considerations
- Managing change
- GPs with specialist interests
- Complementary medicine

THE PARTNERSHIP AGREEMENT

There is usually a clause regarding the division of privately earned money amongst the partners within the practice agreement. Usually, if all the partners agree that a service is to be provided during normal working hours, then the earnings would go to the partnership. If the partner, with the consent of the rest of the partnership, provides the service in the partner's own time, he keeps the earnings but pays the partnership an agreed amount in rent to cover electricity, heating etc.

The question arises: is it ethical that doctors charge their patients for non-GMS treatment provided during the doctor's usual hours of work? Doctors charge their patients for DVLA and insurance medicals, but these are not treatments. Is homeopathy considered a treatment?

THE EVIDENCE BASE FOR HOMEOPATHY

Since 1991 there have been 5 published meta-analyses of homeopathic randomised controlled trials (RCTs), and all conclude that homeopathy has a positive and specific effect beyond that of placebo (Linde K *et al.*, 1997). However, both Linde *et al.* (1997) and the NHS Centre for Reviews and Dissemination at the University of York conclude that there is currently insufficient data to recommend homeopathy as a treatment for any *specific* condition and that more research is needed. Specific evidence does exist for three conditions (hayfever, post-op ileus and rheumatoid arthritis) but limited evidence exists for other conditions (see *Table 3*).

Table 3. *Evidence for effectiveness of homeopathy*

Focused meta-analyses with positive conclusion	At least 2 RCTs showing positive evidence	Single RCTs showing positive evidence
Hayfever Post-op ileus Rheumatoid arthritis	Asthma Childhood diarrhoea Fibrositis Influenza Muscle soreness Otitis media Pain (miscellaneous) Radiotherapy side effects Sprains URTIs	Anxiety ADHD IBS Migraine Osteoarthritis PMS

From: Faculty of Homeopathy (2003) *Homeopathy: a guide for GPs.* HSA Charitable Trust, Luton.

ETHICAL CONSIDERATIONS (using an alternative framework to autonomy, beneficence, non-maleficence and justice):

When introducing a new service, doctors need to ensure that the service offers:

- **appropriateness** – the demand needs to be weighed up against the evidence. Doctors would find it difficult to offer witchcraft even if there was a demand for it! However, there seem to be few negative side effects from homeopathic treatment so offering it in the face of increasing patient demand seems to be appropriate.
- **cost-effectiveness** – 1 in 10 people in the UK visited an alternative practitioner in 2001, which equates to 22 million consultations, that is 8 million more than A and E. The most common conditions for which patients presented were chronic illness, stress-related problems and painful conditions. There is no research data comparing the cost-effectiveness of CAM to conventional treatments, but how cost-effective is conventional medicine for these conditions?
- **acceptability** – 22 million consultations in one year for CAM show that osteopaths, chiropractors, acupuncturists, homeopaths, herbalists, hypnotherapists and reflexologists must be 'acceptable' to the public.
- **patient choice** – 35% of GPs provide simple CAM themselves. Since fundholding ceased, referral to NHS-funded CAM has become more difficult. There are five NHS homeopathic hospitals in the UK, the two biggest being in London and Glasgow. GPs can refer directly to these hospitals under a service agreement or through the Out of Area Treatments arrangement.

MANAGING CHANGE

The partners need to agree:

- Do they want to introduce homeopathy?
- Would patients pay for the service?
- Should the service be offered within partner's hours or in his private time?
- How will the practice know if their patients want it – is there a demand for the service?
- How will the service be evaluated?
- Should it be offered to other practices and will the PCT fund it?

GPs WITH SPECIAL INTERESTS (GPwSIs)

Is your partner interested in becoming a GPwSI in homeopathic medicine? Does he need any specific qualifications before he starts practising? What are the requirements of his medical defence union? Is he intending to further his qualification and how much study time will he require? The Faculty of Homeopathy offers training to doctors. Introductory training will allow the doctor to use a limited number of homeopathic medicines in the treatment of common acute conditions. MFHom is a membership examination and will require more intensive study. See www.trusthomeopathy.org/faculty.

LEARNING POINTS

- There is currently insufficient data to recommend homeopathy
- Specific evidence exists for hayfever, post-op ileus and rheumatoid arthritis
- 1 in 10 people used CAM in 2001
- 35% of GPs provide simple CAM
- Faculty of Homeopathy trains doctors, including GPwSIs

ADDITIONAL INFORMATION

What is homeopathy? It is a system of medicine that stimulates the body's natural immune responses. It works on the principle that 'like treats like', e.g. onion can be used to treat hayfever patients with watery eyes. Homeopathic remedies are known as potencies. They are prepared by serial dilution and succussion (vigorous shaking). The end product is so diluted it is unlikely to contain a single molecule of the active ingredient.

A survey of 1000 patients by health education charity Doctor Patient Partnerships (DPP) found that 71% said they wanted to talk about alternative therapies with pharmacists or doctors but 38% felt most doctors disapproved of such remedies. A poll of 100 GPs found 52% routinely asked patients about their use of complementary medicine.

In November 2004, the RCGP's prescribing spokesman Dr Jim Kennedy described complementary therapies as a 'broad church' – not a replacement for traditional medicine. He said, 'Some of it has an evidence base, some of it doesn't and some is quite frankly dangerous. As doctors, our first priority is always to protect the health of our patients'.

In 1999, in response to evidence of a growing interest amongst patients in the use of complementary therapies, the BMA produced guidance for GPs on referrals to complementary therapists.

The Department of Health website also provides information about the use of complementary and alternative therapies in the NHS. http://www.dh.gov.uk/.

Chiropractic

All chiropractors now have to be registered with the General Chiropractic Council (GCC), which was established in June 2001. The GCC requires practitioners to have completed a four-year course at an accredited chiropractic college.

Osteopathy

All osteopaths must now be registered with the General Osteopathic Council (GOsC), which was set up in May 2000. To be on the GOsC register, osteopaths must have completed a training programme recognised by the Council.

Acupuncture

In 2000, the BMA published *Acupuncture: efficacy, safety and practice*, which recognises the potential benefits of acupuncture in treating certain conditions such as back pain and migraine.

There are several organisations which represent acupuncturists including:

The British Medical Acupuncture Society (BMAS). Full members of the BMAS must be UK-registered doctors and dentists, although associate membership is also open to other health professionals, such as physiotherapists and nurses.

The British Acupuncture Council (BAcC). This is an organisation which accredits institutions providing acupuncture training. The BAcC requires their members to practise traditional forms of diagnosis and acupuncture treatment.

Homeopathy

The Society of Homeopaths is a professional body for non-medical homeopaths. Its members have to have completed a three year full-time (four year part-time) course in homeopathy, in addition to a six-month registration period.

The Faculty of Homeopathy runs postgraduate training courses in homeopathy for doctors, dentists, nurses and other healthcare professionals.

Herbal medicine

The National Institute of Medical Herbalists is the leading organisation for herbalists who prescribe and dispense herbal remedies. Membership of the

Institute is open to those who have completed a three to five year period of training at an accredited college in the UK.

The Medicines and Healthcare Regulatory Agency (MHRA) now publishes Herbal Safety News on its website, providing advice to the public on the safety of different herbal preparations. Some herbal remedies can interact adversely with conventional medicines.

Hypnotherapy

The British Society of Medical and Dental Hypnosis is an organisation of doctors and dentists who practise hypnotherapy as part of their treatment of patients.

RELEVANT LITERATURE

There is a new open access journal from Oxford University Press, *Evidence-based complementary and alternative medicine*: http://www.ecam.oupjournals.org/

Chlamydia screening:

What are the issues raised by screening for chlamydia in primary care?

This question tests communication issues in the context of caring for the wider community.

The question could be answered using three models:

1. Wilson's criteria for screening
2. The ethical model (autonomy, beneficence, non-maleficence and justice)
3. Communication models – one of the consultation models. The Stott and Davis model looks at dealing with four issues within a consultation, namely:
   - management of the presenting problem
   - modification of health-seeking behaviour
   - management of continuing problems
   - opportunist health promotion

   Patients who test positive may respond with embarrassment (fearing a stigma) and anxieties about infertility, contact tracing and the partners' reaction. The clinician needs to be able to sensitively break bad news and advise appropriately.

Wilson's criteria (1966) define the requirements of a robust screening programme:

1. The condition must be:
- Common:
  The national screening pilot found that
    o 14% of under 16 year olds,
    o 11% of 16–19 year olds and
    o 7% of 20–24 year olds were infected.
  It is the commonest curable STD in the UK.
  The natural history of the disease should be known – chlamydia is a sexually transmitted, intracellular, gram-negative infection affecting the genital tract. 70% of infected women and 50% of infected men are asymptomatic (Chief Medical Officer's Report, 2004). Infection may result in severe complications.
- Important: The complications of chlamydia are pelvic inflammatory disease, tubal infertility and ectopic pregnancies. 10–30% of infected women develop PID.
- Diagnosed by acceptable methods: Chlamydia can be diagnosed by two methods:
  o ELISA testing of endocervical and/or urethral swabs. These need to be taken by clinicians. Women find attending a Family Planning Clinic less stigmatising than attending a Genito-urinary medicine clinic (*Sexually Transmitted Infections*, 2003)
  o Polymerase chain reaction or ligase chain reaction on a sample of urine, a vaginal swab or a urethral swab. Studies show that urine sampling is more acceptable than self-taken swabs (Anderson *et al.*, 1998; Ostergaard *et al.*, 1998).

2. There must be a latent interval in which effective interventional treatment is possible. Screening in the USA has led to a 56% reduction in PID. A Swedish study (1998) showed that ectopic pregnancies in 20–24 year olds were more likely to be associated with recent chlamydia infection. Therefore screening for chlamydia and treating it will reduce the incidence of PID and ectopics.

3. Screening must be:

- Cost-effective: The annual costs of chlamydia and its consequences in the UK are estimated to be more than £100 million. Studies from the USA and Sweden have shown that screening for chlamydia is cost-effective (Chief Medical Officer's Report, 2004). Screening can be performed at the time of doing a smear, doing a termination, or seeking gynaecological treatment, thus reducing consultation rates. Postal screening will cost £21 per screening test and £38 per case identified.
- Continuous: The Chief Medical Officer's Report recommends opportunistic (as opposed to continuous) screening – the current programme is focusing on high risk groups e.g. women under 25 years, those seeking termination and prior to insertion of IUDs. There is evidence from the countries which have introduced chlamydia screening that targeted screening of at-risk populations can reduce morbidity.
- Non-invasive and safe: screening is non-invasive and safe.
- Repeatable: it is relatively easy and cheap to repeat the test to confirm the diagnosis.
- Acceptable to patients: urine testing is largely far more acceptable than self-taken urethral or vaginal swabs.
- Highly sensitive (have few false negatives) and highly specific (have few false positives): For LCR, sensitivity is 90% versus 65% for ELISA. Liam Donaldson (CMO) highlighted the clinical governance issue of continuing to use suboptimal tests.
- Easy to interpret: PCR and LCR are relatively easy to interpret. Joint work with the Ministry of Defence intends to develop near patient testing (called NPTgold) which will give a result within one hour of testing.

LEARNING POINTS

- Wilson's criteria
- Tests: ELISA, PCR or LCR
- Screening reduces PID and ectopics
- Cost effective if high risk groups are screened opportunistically
- Near patient testing – NPTgold

ADDITIONAL INFORMATION

Donym S (2004) Sexual health entering primary care: is prevention better than cure? *The Journal of Family Planning and Reproductive Healthcare*, **30**(4), 267.

Over 10% of screening in the pilot programme was done in primary care. However, this depended on the goodwill of GPs. The new GMS contract does provide opportunities to remunerate GPs for opportunistic screening. However, there is debate as to whether sexual health services should be classified as 'essential' or 'enhanced'. Many GPs will argue that it is an enhanced service to ensure that they get paid for providing it. The paymasters will argue against this to contain costs. The obstacles to introducing chlamydia screening into primary care include:

- a lack of resources
- a lack of time
- the issues of contact tracing and partner notification
- the acceptability of the GP-based service to patients. Patients may prefer the anonymity of a GUM clinic
- if GUM clinics and GP practices both offer the service, it is in danger of becoming piecemeal and patients may 'slip through the net'. Who will take responsibility for providing the call and recall service?

Benefits of screening
Screening tests are relatively inexpensive when compared with the treatment of chronic disease or major operations.

A healthy person is screened – disease is picked up at a very early stage when effective, less invasive and life-saving intervention can be offered.

Resources are invested to improve the health of the population as a whole – the service is proactive rather than reactive.

Harms of screening
The total expense of all screening programmes in the UK is considerable (£500 million per annum in 1995 – Bandolier)

A healthy person is invited to be screened – a test that has false positives causes anxiety in a healthy, asymptomatic person who, following the screening test, may be subjected to more invasive definitive testing.

Resources are limited. Are screening programmes cost-effective? Would it not be better to invest the money in treating symptomatic patients, e.g. stroke patients?

McNulty CAM, Freeman E (2004) Barriers to opportunistic chlamydia testing in primary care. *British Journal of General Practice*, **54**(504), 508–514.

This qualitative study based in Herefordshire, Gloucestershire and Avon identified the greatest barriers to opportunistic chlamydia testing and screening in general practice as lack of knowledge of the benefits of testing, when and how to take specimens, lack of time, worries about discussing sexual health, and lack of guidance. Staff felt that any increased testing should be accompanied by clear, concise primary care trust guidance on when and how to test, including how to obtain informed consent and perform contact tracing. The study concluded that efforts to increase chlamydia screening in GP practices should be accompanied by clear guidance and education. Genito-urinary medicine clinics will need to be increased in parallel with testing in primary care to provide appropriate contact tracing and follow-up.

RELEVANT LITERATURE

Anderson B, Ostergaard L, Moller JK, Olesen F (1998) **Home sampling versus conventional contact tracing for detecting Chlamydia trachomatis infection in male partners of infected women: randomised study.** BMJ, **316,** 350–1.

Chief Medical Officer's Expert Advisory Group (2001) **Summary and conclusions of CMO's expert advisory group on Chlamydia.** London: DoH. http://www.dh.gov.uk/assetRoot/04/06/22/64/04062264.pdf

DoH (2004) **The first steps: annual report for the National Chlamydia Screening Programme in England 2003–2004.** http://www.dh.gov.uk/assetRoot/04/09/30/91/04093091.pdf

Oakeshott P, Hay P, Pakianathan M (2004) **Chlamydia screening in primary care.** British Journal of General Practice, **54**(504), 491–493.

Ostergaard L, Anderson B, Olesen F, Moller JK (1998) **Efficacy of home sampling for screening of Chlamydia trachomatis: randomised study.** BMJ, **317,** 26–7.

Wareham NJ and Griffin SJ (2001) **Should we screen for type 2 diabetes? Evaluation against National Screening Committee criteria.** BMJ, **322,** 986–988.

Wilson JMG and Jungner G (1966) **Principles and practice of screening for disease.** WHO.

Cervical screening:
A 28 year old woman on your list repeatedly declines a smear test, saying she is not
sexually active. What would you do?

This question tests the doctor's professional values in the context of caring for patients.

A decision-making model, borrowed from the business world, can be applied to ethical dilemmas in the MRCGP oral examination. The decision-prompting model involves the following steps:

- Recognise the dilemma
- Options – what are your possible options?
- Implication – what are the advantages and disadvantages of each option?
- Choice – which option would you choose?
- Justify – why would you choose this option?
- Check – how will you know that you have made the right choice?

DILEMMA (ethical)

Autonomy

A patient can refuse to have a smear. A health professional needs to explain the reasons for the smear, the advantages (i.e. picking up early dysplasia and cancer) and the disadvantages (discomfort, false positives and negatives). The patient can refuse the treatment and the reasons for her refusal need not be sensible, rational or even well-considered. Being of sound mind, and not being unduly influenced by other parties, she has the right to decide for herself.

Beneficence

A smear has the ability to detect cervical dysplasia at an earlier stage when less invasive treatments can be offered – that is, it has great potential to improve her health outcomes. Screening prevents 1000–4000 deaths per year in the UK from squamous cell carcinoma (www.cancerscreening.nhs.uk/cervical/index.html)

Non-maleficence

Cervical cancer is highest in sexually active women, and those infected with Human Papilloma Virus, especially type 16 and 18.

The Bristol study involving approximately 226 000 women (Raffle et al., 1995) showed that new abnormalities were found in 7% of women; 2.5% had colposcopy. The specificity of cervical screening was not optimal – there was considerable harm from screening. A sexually inactive woman is at lower risk of developing cervical cancer. The patient could have weighed up the risk:benefit ratio and decided against screening. The psychological and social impact of a false positive smear cannot be underestimated.

Target payments for cervical screening were introduced in the UK in 1990. Payments are triggered on reaching 50% or 80% coverage over the last 5 years with the payments for reaching 80% being three times higher. The 80% coverage increased from 53% in 1990 to more than 80% since 1993. There may have been a financial incentive for GPs to provide biased patient information which emphasises the benefits of screening whilst glossing over the risks and side effects. Target payments for screening work against the spirit of enabling women to make an informed choice on whether or not they want to be screened.

Justice
Smear guidelines often lag behind current research. Perhaps the patient may take up the offer of a liquid based cytology screening which is less likely to be reported as 'inadequate'. Pilot studies have shown that the number of inadequate smears was reduced from 9% to 1–2% (Moss *et al.*, 2003).

OPTIONS AND IMPLICATIONS

1. Respect the patient's autonomy. However, the patient must make an informed decision – it is the health care professional's duty to provide adequate information, in language the patient can understand, about the procedure and both the advantages and disadvantages of screening.
2. Ask the patient to make an appointment to see you. The patient may see this as coercion, and legally, the patient's consent should not be unduly influenced by others.
3. Send yearly reminders with up-to-date National Screening Programme leaflets. This allows the patient to make a decision based on the new evidence, and alter her stance accordingly.
4. Remove the patient from your list! The new GMS contract awards 11 Q and O points to practices which achieve 80% coverage. The income generated (approximately £1375 in 2005) can be used to develop further services within the practice for the benefit of all the patients. By removing the patient from your list to achieve target payments, you will be doing the greatest good for the greatest number of patients – using a utilitarianism argument (beware that the RCGP advises against this course of action).

CHOICE

I will send yearly reminders with updated information so that the patient can make an informed decision. I will respect her decision.

JUSTIFY YOUR DECISION

I will respect the patient's autonomy (her right to make informed decisions) over the principles of beneficence and utilitarianism. The GMC's *Good medical practice* states that the care of the patient is the doctor's first concern (patient primacy). The new GMS contract recognises the right of patients to decline screening and awards some Q and O points accordingly.

CHECK AND REFLECT

I would audit the percentage of women who decline the offer of a smear and compare this to the local and national average. Is there something about our practice that is causing women to decline? I would audit the percentage of inadequate smears within the practice – are women declining because we offer a less than optimal service? Do any smear takers need retraining? I would look at the type of patient information that is sent out and ensure that it is simply written, unbiased and up-to-date.

LEARNING POINTS

- A patient has the right to refuse treatment. Her decision is invalid if she was coerced
- The lack of specificity in cervical screening results in too many colposcopies
- Target payments are triggered by reaching 50% and 80% coverage
- Liquid cytology reduces inadequate smears from 9% to 1%
- The GMC's *Good medical practice* emphasises patient primacy

---

RELEVANT LITERATURE

Moss SM, Gray A, Legood R and Henstock E (2003). **Evaluation of HPV/LBC cervical screening pilot studies**. First report to the Department of Health on evaluation of LBC (December 2002, revised Janury 2003). Cancer Screening Evaluation Unit, Sutton.

Muir Gray JA (2004) **New concepts in screening.** British Journal of General Practice, **54**(501), 292–298.

Raffle AE, Alden B and Mackenzie EF (1995). **Detection rates for abnormal cervical smears: what are we screening for?** Lancet, **345**, 1469–73.

This question tests the doctor's consultation skills in the context of caring for patients.

The important features of patient-centred consulting are:

- Understanding the 'whole' person – having a holistic perspective
- Exploring the patient's wants, needs and health beliefs
- Based on a shared understanding of the illness, negotiating a mutually acceptable treatment plan with the patient (concordance).

WHAT IS CONCORDANCE?

Concordance is a shared treatment contract between the prescriber and the patient – the power is shared by the two parties. It differs from compliance where the balance of power lies with the prescriber; the patient being the passive recipient of a treatment plan which is devised by the prescriber in the patient's best interests. The pendulum has now swung away from medical paternalism towards a respect for patient autonomy. In Berne terminology, the relationship is more one of adult–adult than parent–child.

Patients want to make decisions in partnership with doctors. All patients are different and vary in their preference for:

- desiring information – some want direction to alternative sources of information, while others want to know what the doctor thinks is best.
- needing assistance with interpreting the information – some internet users want help with understanding the outcomes of drug trials, while other patients simply want a clarification of what the hospital consultant said.
- help with the final decision-making – some patients want active guidance from their doctors while others wish to make their decisions themselves.

The essence of effective patient-centred consulting is to know the patient well and to facilitate their choices.

Why is patient-centred consulting important?

- Some people argue that it is fashionable. It is in vogue with the RCGP – the marking criteria for the video component award marks for patient-centred doctor behaviour.
- It is part of a national policy as detailed in *Patient partnership: building a collaborative strategy* (NHS Executive, 1996)
- In patient-centred consultations, fewer investigations and referrals are generated (Stewart, 1984).
- Patient-centred consulting achieves better treatment outcomes in the management of chronic diseases (Kaplan *et al.*, 1989).
- Patient-centred consulting improves patient satisfaction – the patients like it! (Howie *et al.*, 1997)

- Patient-centred consulting is achievable – doctors can be trained to consult in this way!

LEARNING POINTS

- Concordance versus compliance
- *Patient partnership: building a collaborative strategy*

If the examiners want to push you further, they will ask you:

- To give instances when it is appropriate to be patient-centred or doctor-centred.
- What are the advantages and disadvantages of patient-centredness or doctor-centredness?
- What influences your decision to consult in a patient-centred manner?
- If faced with a situation when you behaved in a doctor-centred way, in six months, how will you know if you had made the right choice?

ADDITIONAL INFORMATION

From Gamey G. Looking after patients who won't look after themselves. *studentBMJ*: http://www.studentbmj.com/back_issues/0200/education/17.html

Gamey writes: 'As doctors, we tend to like those patients who do what they are told. Such patients are "complying" with our advice. But this kind of paternalistic relationship is outdated and unhelpful. The patient's view of the world – based on experience, culture, family history, and personality – may be different from ours. If we see this as an obstacle to be overcome at all costs we will alienate our patients and they will continue to make unhealthy choices. Encounters between doctors and patients entail the bringing together of often conflicting explanatory systems about illness and health, and negotiation is the key to a "successful" outcome. We should try to build an honest and open therapeutic alliance with our patients, sharing our own thoughts and beliefs with them, to reach a mutually respectful agreement. This model of working is called "concordance" and it has replaced the term "compliance".'

Elwyn G (2004) Arriving at the postmodern medical consultation. *European Journal of General Practice*, **10**(3), 93–7.

The analysis of the medical consultation is characterised by mainly prescriptive attempts to recommend 'best practice'. As the role of the individual in society has gained prominence, the power relationships in medical practice have had to change to reflect the increasing recognition of autonomy and self-determination. Medical discourse is at a junction, having to relinquish authoritarianism and grapple with the concept of sharing information and decisions in an area where complex and uncertain data exist, albeit often without full disclosure. The concept of postmodernism fits well with the idea that the consultation between doctors and patients is increasingly becoming a contested space that occupies multiple voices, such as that of the media, the pharmaceutical industry, government-led guidelines and that of the profession. Creating the circumstances and the means for creating an effective dialogue in the postmodern consultation is the prime task for physicians.

Morgan ED, Pasquarella M *et al.* (2004) Continuity of care and patient satisfaction in a family practice clinic. *Journal of the American Board of Family Practitioners*, **17**(5), 341–6.

Continuity of care is important to general practice. This American study surveyed the patients of a military practice over a period of one week. The response rate was 68.3%. Responders were not more likely to be seeing their own doctor. Regression analysis revealed that:

- 12% of patient satisfaction was associated with long-term continuity rates,
- 23% by satisfaction with the doctor, and
- 17% by how easy it was to make the appointment.
- A subset of patients (13%) values choice of appointment time or choice of other doctors over continuity of care.

The study concluded that patient satisfaction is associated with continuity, especially for high clinic users. Although continuity is important, a subset of patients values the ability to see other doctors and to change doctors.

RELEVANT LITERATURE

Howie JG, Heaney DJ, Maxwell M (1997) **Measuring quality in general practice. Pilot study of a needs, process and outcome measure.** *Occasional Paper Royal College General Practice.* 1997 Feb, **(75)**:i–xii, 1–32.
Kaplan SH, Greenfield S and Ware JE (1989) **Assessing the effects of physician–patient interactions on the outcomes of chronic disease.** *Med Care,* **27**, 5110–27.
Kinnersley P, Peters JT, and Harvey I (1999) **The patient-centredness of consultations and outcome in Primary Care.** *Br J Gen Pract,* **49**(446), 711–716.
Stewart MA (1984) **What is a successful doctor–patient interview? A study of interactions and outcomes.** *Social Science and Medicine,* **19**, 167–75.
Improve your communication skills: http://www.skillscascade.com/handouts.htm
In particular, see http://www.skillscascade.com/files/commresearch.htm and http://www.skillscascade.com/files/research.htm
From King's Fund: http://www.kingsfund.org.uk/pdf/duncanmemorial.pdf

A 76 year old man (Mr B) was recently informed by the respiratory physicians that he has inoperable lung cancer. He comes to see you saying that he did not fully understand what the hospital doctors told him. You have the test results from the hospital. Discuss how you would break bad news to patients.

This question tests the doctor's ability to communicate well with patients to improve their care.

As this is likely to be a difficult situation, I would use Roger Neighbour's consultation model to structure my actions. This is not a step-wise process – I would 'connect' throughout the consultation. Alternatively, I can structure my consultation using the SPIKES approach: Setting up, Perception, Invitation, Knowledge, Emotions, Strategy and summary.

CONNECT

- Eye contact; warm welcome; empathy – acknowledge the patient's feelings throughout the consultation; touch; privacy; appropriate use of silence.
- Remark upon his expression / movements / state of agitation (non-verbal cues), for example, 'Mr B, you look upset today.'
- Ask open questions to establish his agenda. Has he come to confirm the specialist's diagnosis, or is he querying the inoperability of the cancer? – i.e. establish his ideas, concerns and expectations.
- Establish what he understands, and what he wants to know. The vast majority of patients prefer to be privy to their diagnosis of cancer. Disclosure allows the patient to make informed decisions, like making a will. Inadequate support is provided when the family and doctor hide the diagnosis from the patient. Beware of breaking confidentiality by discussing the issue with the family instead of the patient.

SUMMARISE

- Use language the patient understands (jargon-free).
- Use the patient's own words. 'Am I right in thinking that you were confused about what the hospital doctors meant by *a shadow on the lung*? Are you also worried about them saying it was inoperable?'
- Patients who are given bad news often do not retain much factual information beyond the initial shock. He may need a careful explanation of what the shadow on the lung is. He may need prompting about his fears. Is he looking to confirm his fears? Use simple language, be tactful, sensitive, but be honest. He needs help in dealing with the emotions such news can cause. Give him time and space to vent his emotions.

HANDOVER

- Confirm that he has understood the diagnosis. Ask him what he would tell his wife – ask him to repeat the information back to you.
- Give him permission to return with further questions: 'People often walk out of a doctor's surgery and think of all sorts of questions that they should have asked. If this happens to you, please come back and ask me these questions.'
- If the patient is mentally prepared, you can outline a management plan, but if not, this can wait until follow-up.

SAFETY NET

- Arrange follow-up, either formally, or leave it up to the patient. For example, 'Mr B, we discussed a huge amount of information, most of it very upsetting. I need to talk to you again. Would you mind seeing me, perhaps with your wife, in a few days' time, or I could visit you at home?'
- At follow-up, check the patient's understanding and address further concerns. Introduce the liaison services (Marie Curie and day-service hospice care). Provide support to the patient and his family. Social benefits may also need to be discussed.

HOUSEKEEPING

- Acknowledge your own feelings: long, difficult, emotionally draining consultation.
- Inform members of PHCT so that they are aware of and sensitive to the patient and family's recent shock.
- Discuss at next significant event meeting.

LEARNING POINTS

- SPIKES
- Don't hide the diagnosis from patient – it creates a conspiracy of silence
- Information in moderation
- Liaison services (Marie Curie and day-service hospice care)
- Significant event meeting – morbidity and mortality indices.

If the examiner wants to push you further, he will ask:

- Name the different ways in which a doctor can break bad news.
- What are the possible advantages and disadvantages of each of these methods?
- Which method(s) will you choose and why?
- On reviewing your work in six months, how would you know if you had broken the bad news well?

ADDITIONAL INFORMATION

The SPIKES approach to breaking bad news
Baile *et al.* (2000) coined the mnemonic SPIKES

- **S**etting up: allow sufficient time, privacy and minimise interruptions.
- **P**erception: what the patient knows (his perceptions), so that you tailor your explanation according to his understanding.
- **I**nvitation: get the patient's permission to break the bad news and ask if the patient wants basic information or a detailed disclosure.
- **K**nowledge: give the patient sufficient information, using jargon-free language to enable him to make informed decisions.
- **E**motions: acknowledge the patient's feelings. Use silence – allow the patient to vent his emotions.
- **S**trategy and summary: summarise the information discussed, check comprehension, provide written plans / information and make follow-up arrangements.

This approach is intended to help physicians break bad news to patients in a straightforward and empathic manner.

Elisabeth Kübler-Ross theory
Elisabeth Kübler-Ross (1969) wrote that people pass through five stages of coping with dying. Not everyone goes through each stage and in the same order.

1. Denial and isolation: this is usually a temporary shock response to bad news.
2. Anger: 'Why me?'
3. Bargaining: this often occurs between patient and God – 'If only I could live to see...'
4. Depression: mourning for losses.
5. Acceptance: the person accepts that death is inevitable.

RELEVANT LITERATURE

Baile WF, Buckman R, Lenzi R *et al.* (2000) **SPIKES – A six-step protocol for delivering bad news: application to the patient with cancer.** *Oncologist*, **5(4)**, 302–11.

Kübler-Ross E (1969) **On death and dying.** *Springer*, New York.

Mueller PS (2002) **Breaking bad news to patients: the SPIKES approach can make this difficult task easier.** *Postgraduate Medicine Online*, **112**(3) http://www.postgradmed.com/issues/2002/09_02/editorial_sep.htm

http://www.skillscascade.com/badnews.htm: preparation; beginning the session / setting the scene; sharing the information; being sensitive to the patient; planning and support; follow-up and closing.

A useful summary from an Australian website: http://www.medicineau.net.au/clinical/palliativecare/palliativec1623.html

Your practice looks after the families of a nearby military establishment. The midwife asks Mrs H-T, the 36 year old wife of a high ranking officer, to see you. The midwife's computer notes state that she saw bruises on Mrs H-T's arms and she suspects domestic violence. What would you do for Mrs H-T?

This question tests the doctor's communication skills in the context of caring for patients, as well as his personal responsibility in caring for vulnerable people.

In answering this question, two approaches spring to mind.

- The question can be considered in terms of a consultation model which is useful for navigating challenging patient–doctor dynamics, or
- In ethical terms, the pros and cons of each action may be considered before deciding on a morally justifiable course of action.

Any of the consultation models can be applied to this scenario. Balint's work from the 1950s highlights important concepts which assist the doctor in dealing with emotionally challenging consultations. Balint (1957) suggested that specific training is needed to change the doctor's behaviour so that he can become more sensitive to the patient. Important concepts are:

1. **The doctor as a drug**

Domestic violence in pregnancy is more common than pre-eclampsia, gestational diabetes and twin pregnancies (DoH, 2000). Health professionals will fail in their responsibilities if they do not ask about domestic violence. The dilemma with suspected cases of domestic violence is the timing of the question. Because domestic violence is so easy to miss, some people advocate that routine screening should occur. On the other hand, some groups, such as the RCGP, are of the opinion that routine screening is intrusive and GPs should wait for women to volunteer their concerns. However, in the above scenario, it is not a question of screening. The patient was referred by a fellow professional on the suspicion of domestic violence – this cannot be ignored. Doctors have a professional responsibility to take a proactive approach and be instrumental in their treatment of patients – the doctor as a drug.

Balint wrote that although the doctor is an important drug, no guidance exists as to when he should be prescribed. In the above scenario, a significant health problem may exist. If the doctor:

- does not 'prescribe himself', i.e. does not ask about the bruises and raise the midwife's concerns, harm may occur to Mrs H-T and her unborn child.
- 'prescribes himself', i.e. asks about the bruises, he risks offending Mrs H-T. Of women visiting their GP, at least 20% said that they would object to being asked about abuse or violence in their relationship if they had come about something else (Richardson *et al.*, 2002). If the doctor asks Mrs H-T in the presence of the perpetrator, the violence may escalate and the doctor could put Mrs H-T seriously at risk.

2. The collusion of anonymity

The midwife is an independent practitioner and had the opportunity to raise the concerns about domestic violence herself. By referring the patient, she has transferred the clinical responsibility to the GP. The GP could refer the patient to the obstetricians; however, in passing the responsibility from one speciality to another, nobody is taking responsibility for the patient – this is termed the collusion of anonymity. Some GPs are wary of taking responsibility for a social problem – they believe that their job is to signpost patients to the appropriate welfare services, such as Women's Aid (Shakespeare, 2002). However, Judge Mornington, who founded 'Raising the Standards', an inter-governmental initiative on domestic violence, is of the opinion that:

- the medical profession has a moral duty to take responsibility and that it has badly failed victims in the past.
- doctors will be called to court more often and need to accurately record domestic violence in writing or by taking photographs.
- doctors need to address the cause rather than continually treat symptoms. Vast amounts of time are wasted because doctors fail to identify the hidden agendas of patients who repeatedly present with somatic symptoms such as headaches, anxiety, insomnia, weight loss and repeated 'accidental' injuries.

3. The mutual investment fund

This term was coined by Balint to describe the shared experiences and trust that the GP and patient accumulate over many years. The GP and Mrs H-T may have established a good doctor–patient relationship over many years, hence the GP may think the probability of domestic violence is slim and that the junior midwife's suspicions are ill-founded. However, within this relationship of trust, the GP could sensitively raise the concerns without fear of jeopardizing the relationship. Most women will not be offended by a sensitive and non-judgemental enquiry. In fact, many women do not understand the failure of health professionals to ask in depth about the cause of their injuries or health problems (Davidson *et al.*, 2000).

What would you do?

I would ask Mrs H-T about her bruises because:

- I have a moral duty to Mrs H-T, her unborn child and her other children to raise the issue and to act if necessary. Domestic violence and child abuse often co-exist (RCGP, 2002).
- As Mrs H-T's GP, I have a professional obligation under the GMC's *Good medical practice.*
  - I must make the care of the patient my first concern.
  - However, I also need to respect the rights of patients to make their own decisions regarding their care. It is not my job to tell Mrs H-T what to do. At the very least, I can provide her with information on where to go for help (Women's Aid Group, police community safety unit, victim support).
  - In addition, I need to respect and protect Mrs H-T's confidential information. By ensuring that Mrs H-T understands the confidential

nature of the consultation, I might encourage her to discuss her fears more openly. If this is a case of domestic violence, any notes I make may be used as evidence in court. I will document my findings carefully. I will also keep these notes separately from any notes held by the patient (such as her pregnancy book) to which the perpetrator may have access. I will obtain the patient's consent before releasing any of her medical information to other professionals or health care agencies who may become involved.

○ On the other hand, confidentiality must be balanced against the public interests in protecting vulnerable people, such as Mrs H-T's children, from serious harm. Thus, in rare cases, a breach of confidentiality may be justified if Mrs H-T's silence puts her children at risk and if I cannot persuade her to make a voluntary disclosure (BMA, 1994). I will follow child protection guidelines if I believe that her children are at risk.

● I have a good relationship with Mrs H-T and my sensitive enquiry is unlikely to jeopardize the trust within our relationship. I could ask the question indirectly, such as, 'Is everything all right at home?'

● In certain situations it may be more appropriate to ask direct questions, such as, 'I don't wish to cause you any offence, but we know that one in four women experiences violence at home at some time during their lives. I noticed that you have a number of bruises. Could you tell me how you got those bruises?'

I would not ask Mrs H-T about her bruises because:
● I would respect her autonomy and wait for Mrs H-T to broach the subject when she felt ready to do so. I would be sensitive, approachable and non-judgemental so that she would feel comfortable seeking help when she requires it. She is currently taking responsibility for her own health and that of her children and is very likely to know which decisions are best for her. My well-intended interference may at best be perceived as meddling, and at worst may scare the patient away.

● I know the patient well enough to be confident that domestic violence is not the cause of her bruises. If I truly suspected a problem, I would tackle it. In this instance, it is my considered professional opinion that a problem does not exist, and I am not hiding a lack of time, skill, training or knowledge behind this stance. Mrs H-T has not previously presented in a way that has aroused my suspicions:

○ She does not make frequent appointments for vague symptoms.

○ She does not frequently miss appointments.

○ She has not had any injuries which seem inconsistent with the explanation given, such as falls or walking into doors.

○ She does not have any evidence of multiple injuries at different stages of healing.

○ She does not appear to be excessively frightened, anxious or distressed.

○ She does not have a psychiatric history or a drug or alcohol problem.

○ She is not always accompanied by her partner when she consults.

○ She does not seem to be afraid of her partner, and her partner does not appear to be aggressive or overly dominant.

○ She does not have a history of repeated miscarriages or terminations of pregnancy.

• There is the risk of converting a social issue into a medical problem. General practice can support people during difficult times but it is for the welfare agencies to co-ordinate practical management. My responsibility is to signpost patients appropriately and to work closely with these agencies. By giving Mrs H-T a leaflet on pregnancy care, which includes information on how to access agencies that deal with domestic violence, I have signposted appropriately. (Beware that this stance is not supported by the DoH and BMA – see below).

LEARNING POINTS

- Balint terminology: the doctor as a drug, the collusion of anonymity, the mutual investment fund
- Judge Mornington founded 'Raising the Standards'
- Domestic violence and child abuse often co-exist
- Signposting to Social Services

ADDITIONAL INFORMATION

Judy Shakespeare and Leslie Davidson (2002) *Domestic violence in families with children: Guidance for primary health care professionals*. RCGP, London.

- Domestic violence and child abuse often co-exist. If you find one of these, evaluate the family for the other.
- Managing these situations is complex. It may help to share the decision-making process with other members of your team, or the 'named' doctor or nurse for child protection in your PCT.
- Make a risk assessment for the child. Is the child at risk of significant harm from either parent?
- Support for a non-abusive parent will usually help promote the welfare of the abused parent and her child(ren).
- Document carefully, but keep records about domestic violence and child abuse safely and confidentially.
- Recognise your responsibility to contribute to inter-agency processes, such as Child Protection Conferences.
- Consider whether you can continue to care for the perpetrator of domestic violence and child abuse as well as the victims.
- Since domestic violence is so prevalent it is possible that a member of every practice is experiencing (or perpetrating) domestic violence. Practices need to consider the challenges this brings to an affected individual.

DoH (2000) *Domestic violence: a resource manual for healthcare professionals* states that:

The term 'domestic violence' describes the continuum of behaviour ranging from verbal assault, through threats and intimidation, manipulative behaviour, physical and sexual assault, to rape and even homicide. Those who experience domestic violence often keep it to themselves because:

- they are ashamed of, and embarrassed by what is happening to them;
- they are unsure of where they can go and what help they can get, and
- they are fearful of doing anything which might make the situation worse.

The impact of the violence on the individual's health and well-being is substantial: anxiety, depression, post-traumatic stress and suicide attempts are higher amongst those who are abused. It is not acceptable simply to assume that someone else, such as Social Services or the police, will do something. Those who are being abused may not want the statutory services to become involved, and may prefer to be seen in the NHS. The NHS may be perceived to be less stigmatising than the other services. The NHS should address the underlying causes of the violence and not just deal with the physical and mental consequences of the violence.

23% of women between the ages of 16 and 59 and 15% of men have been assaulted by a current or former partner. Every week in the UK, two women are killed by current or former partners. Domestic violence occurs at similar prevalence among people of all income levels, and among people from white, black and ethnic minority backgrounds. Women with few financial resources face particular difficulty in accessing protection. Women from black and ethnic minorities may face additional challenges, such as racism, when approaching certain institutions and services.

Pregnancy can be a trigger for domestic violence to begin or to intensify, putting both the woman and her unborn child at risk. In all contact with women who have experienced domestic violence, health professionals need to ask themselves, 'Will my intervention leave this woman and her children in greater safety or in greater danger?' Abused women feel ashamed, humiliated, frightened and prone to blaming themselves. Professionals have a duty to treat people with dignity, to help empower them and to maintain their confidentiality. Scepticism from the healthcare professional could drive the woman back into her isolated and violent situation.

Child protection and confidentiality from: http://www.medicalprotection.org/ Medical/United_Kingdom/Publications/Factsheets/factsheet_child.aspx) accessed Nov 2004

Doctors dealing with child protection issues are frequently confronted by conflicts between the need to share information and the rules governing confidentiality, and their professional duties to different patients often within the same family.

- The doctor's first duty is to act in the best interests of the child. Where there is a conflict between parents and child and child and others, the child's needs are paramount.

- Where there are reasonable grounds to believe a child is at risk of significant harm, the facts should be reported to Social Services.
- Primary Care Trusts, NHS Trusts and health authorities have a statutory duty, effected through their employees, to assist Social Services, making enquiries under the Children Act.
- Where consent to disclosure is refused by an apparently competent child, disclosure may still be appropriate if refusal results from duress, fear or the circumstantial pressures upon the child.
- Where consent to disclosure is refused by an adult, relevant disclosure may be necessary in order to protect the best interests of the child and may be justifiable on those grounds.
- All decisions and the reasoning behind them should be thoroughly documented.

RELEVANT LITERATURE

Balint M (1957) **The doctor, his patient and the illness.** *Pitman*, London.

BMA (1998) **Domestic violence: a health issue?**

Davidson LL, Grisso JA, Garcia-Moreno C, Garcia J, King VJ, and Marchant S (2000) **Training programs for healthcare professionals in domestic violence.** *J Women's Health Gender Based Med*, **10**, 953–969.

DoH (2000) **Domestic violence: a resource manual for healthcare professions.** HMSO, London.

Goodyear-Smith F and Arroll B (2004) Screening for domestic violence in general practice: a way forward? *British Journal of General Practice*, **53**(492), 515–518.

Heath I (1998) **Domestic violence: the general practitioner's role.** RCGP, London. www.domesticviolencedata.org

Richardson JR, Feder G, and Coid J (2002) **Domestic violence affects women more than men.** *BMJ*, **325**, 779.

Shakespeare J and Davidson L (2002) **Domestic violence in families with children. Guidance for primary health care professionals.** *RCGP*, London.

Asking women about domestic abuse http://www.bmjlearning.com/planrecord/servlet/ResourceSearchServlet?keyWord=Read%2C+reflect%2C+respondandresourceId=5003147andviewResource=

Teenagers and confidentiality:
A 15 year old patient attends complaining of a wart on his penis. It transpires that he is having a relationship with his 32 year old female teacher. What would you do?

This question tests a doctor's personal responsibility to society as well as his/her communication skills in the context of caring for patients.

A decision-making model, borrowed from the business world, can be applied to ethical dilemmas in the MRCGP oral examination. The decision-prompting model involves the following steps:

- Recognise the dilemma
- Options – what are your possible options?
- Implication – what are the advantages and disadvantages of each option?
- Choice – which option would you choose?
- Justify – why would you choose this option?
- Check – how will you know that you have made the right choice?

RECOGNISE THE DILEMMA

This is an ethical and medico-legal dilemma: the conflicting issues here are the patient's autonomy (the right to have sex with a consenting partner) versus beneficence (the doctor should be acting in the best interests of an underage and vulnerable child). There is also the duty of confidentiality owed to the patient, versus breaking confidentiality to preserve the public interest in protecting the vulnerable.

Young people can legally consent to heterosexual and homosexual sex from the age of 16 years (Sexual Offences Amendment Act, 2000). However, one in four women and one in three men say they had sexual intercourse before the age of 16. The legal position does not mirror the social reality.

- In the above case, a sexual relationship between a 15 year old and a 32 year old is illegal (the minor is below the age of consent).
- In addition, the relationship between teacher and student is based on trust (similar to the relationship between a doctor and his patient). Turning a professional relationship into a sexual relationship violates the trust within the relationship. Even if both parties were consenting, the sexual relationship between teachers and their students can never be considered truly mutual and based on an equal footing; it would always be viewed to some extent as an abuse of the teacher's position of trust.
- If the doctor maintains the patient's confidentiality, is he colluding with the teacher who is abusing her position of power and trust?
- If the doctor breaks the patient's confidentiality, is he sending out a message to teenagers that doctors cannot be trusted to maintain their confidentiality? This message discourages teenagers from seeking medical advice, puts them at risk of teenage pregnancy and sexually transmitted disease, and

discourages vulnerable patients from seeking support in the future. The trust within the patient–doctor relationship is lost.

OPTIONS AND IMPLICATIONS

1. Refer to GUM clinic
Advantages: The wart will be treated and screening for other sexually transmitted diseases will be offered. The doctor transfers responsibility for the ethical dilemma to clinicians who are better trained to deal with these issues – a better service is offered. The trust within the GP–patient relationship is maintained.
Disadvantages: Transferring responsibility to the GUM clinic may be seen as 'passing the buck' or as a 'collusion of anonymity' (Balint). The patient may feel daunted and stigmatised by the prospect of going to a GUM clinic. There may be practical difficulties in accessing the GUM clinic – it may be a bus ride away.

2. Treat the wart without addressing the ethical issues
Advantages: The patient's expectations of the consultation are met. The doctor is approachable and non-judgemental and the patient may feel more comfortable in returning to the doctor to discuss other sensitive issues. Doctor–patient trust is maintained.
Disadvantages: The doctor is seen as potentially colluding with the teacher who is abusing her position of trust and breaking the law. The doctor is not fulfilling his moral and professional duty to society in protecting the interests of the socially vulnerable.

3. Treat the wart and advise the patient to consider the legal and moral aspects of his behaviour
Advantages: The doctor assesses whether the minor is being coerced within the relationship – if coercion (i.e. rape or sexual abuse) is occurring, then Child Protection procedures need to be followed. Social Services need to be contacted. If coercion is not occurring, is the minor competent – does he understand the consequences of his actions? How would he feel if his 15 year old sister had a relationship with her 32 year old male teacher? Does he understand that society has rules against teacher–student relationships to protect the student from being taken advantage of? By informing him of the wider implications of his actions, he can then decide on the moral course of action for himself – you are furthering his autonomy. You can make a reasonable effort to persuade him against having a relationship (especially one that has already harmed his health) but you reassure him that you will not break his confidentiality by approaching the school or his parents. You stress that your door is always open and that he may return to discuss the issue further at a later date. You have respected his autonomy, you have maintained your doctor–patient relationship and you have not broken confidentiality, thus presenting general practice as a teenage-friendly service.
Disadvantages: By placing such emphasis on respecting the patient's autonomy,

you can be accused of allowing a system of abuse to go unchallenged. Your decision to keep quiet can be construed as not wanting to get involved and not wanting to make waves.

4. Treat the wart and contact your medical defence union
Advantages: You will act once you have been advised about the correct medico-legal course of action.
Disadvantages: It may be difficult to contact the patient once he has left the surgery and you may have missed your opportunity to act.

5. Treat the wart and inform Social Services / his school / his parents
Advantages: You are discharging your responsibility to society by informing the relevant agencies so that an investigation of the teacher's alleged misconduct can occur.
Disadvantages: You have breached confidentiality and potentially damaged your relationship of trust with your patient. If his allegations were factually incorrect, you have potentially destroyed a teacher's position within her school and community and possibly blighted her career. You have also sent a message to young people that you will not always respect their confidentiality. Various surveys have estimated that at least 25% of teenagers do not believe that their consultation will be confidential. Teenagers will be less likely to consult and this may have an adverse effect on teenage pregnancy and STD rates. Breaching confidentiality to stop potential abuse may have resulted in greater harm to teenage health in the long run.

CHOICE AND JUSTIFY

There is no right answer. One way in which the question can be answered is listed below.

- I would give the patient the option of treating the wart in surgery or at the GUM clinic.
- I would offer the patient screening for further STDs.
- I would offer contact tracing.
- I would inform him early in the consultation that I am obliged to pass on any information that he volunteers if I strongly believe that he is at risk – i.e. I am obliged to contact Social Services if I felt he was being abused or coerced. This informs the patient of my legal and ethical responsibility and advises him that confidentiality can be broken under certain circumstances. If he then chooses to disclose information, he is aware that the information may be passed on.
- If I believe that he is in a consensual adult relationship, I would advise him about his sexual health, his teacher's professional and legal obligations and ask him to pursue a course that he is morally comfortable with.
- I would contact my medical defence union after the consultation and consider their advice.
- Unless there was a Child Protection issue, I would not breach confidentiality because:

- ○ I would respect the competent teenager's autonomy.
- ○ I would maintain a trusting doctor–patient relationship so that he would feel comfortable in consulting me at a future date.
- ○ I would want to send out a message to other teenagers that I am a GP that can be trusted to respect their confidences and to put their needs first. This will make me more effective in dealing with the issues of teenage pregnancy and the growing epidemic of teenage STDs.

CHECK

Having made a decision that my duty as a doctor is to my teenage patients and not to police the local schools, I would hope to see:

- my patient returning to see me in the future and that he trusts me enough to discuss sensitive issues.
- teenagers continuing to consult my practice.

I would discuss this case at a significant event meeting in the partnership, and would hope that there were no further cases of teacher–student relationships within the practice.

LEARNING POINTS

- Sexual Offences Amendment Act, 2000 – the age of consent is 16
- 'Collusion of anonymity' (Balint)
- 25% of teenagers do not believe that their consultation will be confidential
- Autonomy versus beneficence
- The duty of confidentiality owed to the patient, to preserve the trusting doctor–patient relationship, versus breaking the duty of confidentiality to preserve the public interest in stopping potential abuse

---

ADDITIONAL INFORMATION

When confronted with questions on teenage consent and confidentiality, the Fraser guidelines should be applied. The arguments underlying the Fraser guidelines which are based on the case of *Gillick* v. *West Norfolk and Wisbech Area Health Authority* (1984) are:

- Sociologically, contraception is preferable to abortion.
- Refusal to supply contraception to minors is unlikely to deter those who want sexual intercourse. On this basis, the doctor who supplies contraceptives to a girl under the age of 16 without parental consent is performing a duty to society.

- On the other hand, parents have a right to know what is happening to their children and should ideally give consent to medical treatment irrespective of the minor's capacity to understand the treatment and its implications.

Lord Fraser's five criteria for a minor to consent to contraception without the consent of her parents are:

1. She understands the advice and is competent to consent to treatment.
2. She is encouraged to inform her parents or guardians.
3. She is likely to commence or continue sexual activity with or without contraception.
4. Her physical or mental health will suffer if she does not receive contraceptive advice or supplies.
5. Providing contraception is in her best interests.

RELEVANT LITERATURE

Balint M (1957) **The doctor, his patient and the illness.** *Pitman*, London.

DoH (2001). The Health and Social Care Act 2001: Section 60 and 61. Background information. *Patient Confidentiality*

GMC (2000) **Protecting and providing information.** *BMA*, London. Paragraphs 34 and 35.

Mason JK (2000) **The legal aspects and implications of risk assessment.** *Medical law review*, **8**(69), 106–16.

Neuberger J (2001) **The educated patient: new challenges for the medical profession.** *Journal of internal medicine*, **249,** 41–5.

Sculpher *et al.* (2002) **Shared treatment decision making in a collectively funded health care system: possible conflicts and some potential solutions.** *Social Science and Medicine*, **54**(9), 1369–77.

www.info.doh.gov.uk/tpu/tpu.nsf

Mr McDonald is a 46 year old self employed electrician. He has had well-controlled epilepsy for many years, but unfortunately has recently suffered a seizure. You have advised him to inform the DVLA and to stop driving. You see him driving into the practice car park to collect his medication. What would you do?

This question tests a doctor's personal responsibility to society as well as his communication skills in the context of caring for patients.

The ethical dilemma here is the conflict in interest between the doctor's duty to his patient versus his duty to society. An ethical model can be applied to the above scenario.

Autonomy: The patient has been warned of the risk of sudden incapacitation as a result of his epilepsy. He was made aware of the possible harm to himself and to others including family members and fellow road users. The patient is self-employed and not being able to drive could adversely affect his income and reputation. He has probably weighed up the risks and benefits of not driving and has decided, against medical advice, to continue driving. A competent patient has the right to refuse medical advice – the patient is expressing his autonomy. However, in this case his personal interest needs to be weighed against the public interest in having safe road-users – his expression of autonomy conflicts with society's sense of utilitarianism.

Utilitarianism: states that an action is right if it promotes the best consequences – the greatest good or happiness for the greatest number. If Mr McDonald has a seizure while driving, it could kill or injure many.

Beneficence: The doctor should try to do the best for his patient and to promote his best interests. It is in Mr McDonald's best interests to stop driving because he may die on the roads, he may be responsible for manslaughter and he may face criminal proceedings should an accident occur. The question is, what is the likelihood of Mr McDonald actually having a second seizure? The risk of having a second seizure will decrease with time to a point at which his risk of sudden incapacitation is deemed negligible. The DVLA sets this point at the one year mark – Mr McDonald can legally drive if he remains fit-free for one year (Road Traffic Act, 1988). If he holds an HGV licence, he can drive vocationally only if he remains fit-free and off treatment for 10 years.

The doctor tries to do the best for his patient by:

- explaining to him in simple language the importance of not driving and the risk to himself and others.
- informing the patient of the patient's legal duty to inform the DVLA.
- making all reasonable efforts to encourage the patient to disclose the information voluntarily.
- unless it is a situation of great urgency, giving the patient time in which to act responsibly.

- informing the patient (if the previous measures are ineffective) of the doctor's intention to disclose the information to the DVLA medical advisor. The doctor should try to seek the patient's consent for this disclosure.

Should the patient fail to consent to disclosure, the doctor should seek the advice of his defence body. If the doctor does not disclose and serious harm results, then he is open to a charge of negligence.

Non-maleficence: Patients know that their disclosures to health care professionals are treated confidentially. If medical confidentiality is regularly breached, then patients lose trust in the profession. This may prevent patients from seeking appropriate medical treatment at times of need, e.g. patients with sexually transmitted diseases may be reluctant to seek medical attention if they feel their confidentiality will not be respected. Therefore there is a public interest to maintain confidentiality to protect society. The public interest in maintaining confidence needs to be weighed up, or balanced, with the countervailing public interest favouring disclosure, such as protecting the public from dangerous drivers.

What would you do?
- Inform the patient again of the risks of driving so soon after a seizure.
- Inform the patient that he has a legal obligation to inform the DVLA.
- If he refuses to inform the DVLA, make every reasonable effort to persuade him to stop driving.
- If he continues to refuse, inform him of your intention to inform the DVLA – try to do so with his consent.
- Pass on the relevant (minimal) information to the DVLA's medical advisor.
- Try to maintain a good working relationship with the patient if at all possible!

LEARNING POINTS

- Risk of sudden incapacitation
- Charge of negligence
- DVLA medical advisors

ADDITIONAL INFORMATION

When can confidentiality be breached?
The GMC does provide guidance about the disclosure of patient information, and its ethical standards largely reflect the legal standards. Exceptions to the duty of confidence exist in six main areas:

- **Consent:** the patient consents to the disclosure of information. Consent implies more than agreement, and takes into account competence, understanding and voluntary participation. Consent can be expressed (explicit) or implied (implicit). Implied consent means that the patient is aware of the practice of disclosure and has the option of opting out, as in HIV testing of pregnant women.

- **Public interest:** the public interest in maintaining confidence needs to be weighed up, or balanced, with the countervailing public interest favouring disclosure, such as protecting the public purse from people trying to defraud the health service, or protecting the public from dangerous people, such as psychotics wielding a knife or HIV-infected patients knowingly having unprotected sex with partners who are unaware of their HIV status.

- **Teaching, research and clinical audit:** Patients have a choice (expressed as consent) in participating in research and medical student training. Research benefits society. The rights of patients not wanting to participate in research, such as inclusion within cancer registries, needs to be weighed against the necessity of medical research and its benefit to society – individual personal interest versus public interest.

- **Management and NHS administrative purposes:** There is a public interest in spending public money efficiently in the NHS, and financial auditors need access to some patient information to monitor NHS spending. National Health Service Act 1977 provides the statutory backing for financial auditors to access patient information.

- **Genetics:** The information obtained from the genetic testing of an individual has consequences not only for that individual, but also for other family members. The duty to the individual has to be balanced with a duty to other family members, and the possible impact of the genetic information on their health decisions (particularly with regard to exercising reproductive choice, or entering screening programmes).

- **Under particular statutes:**
  - The Abortion Regulations 1999
  - Public Health (Control of Disease) Act 1984
  - National Health Service (Venereal Diseases) Regulations 1974
  - Police and Criminal Evidence Act 1984
  - Health Act 1999
  - Health Service Commissioner Act 1993

RELEVANT LITERATURE

BMA (1998) **Human genetics: choice and responsibility.** BMA, London.
Case P (2003) **Confidence matters: the rise and fall of informational autonomy in medical law.** Medical Law Review, **11**, 208–29.
Department of Health (1996) **The protection and use of patient information.**
General Practitioners Committee (2002) **Good medical practice for general practitioners.** Royal College of General Practitioners, London.
GMC (2000) **Protecting and providing information.** Paragraphs 34 and 35. BMA, London.

Kennedy and Grubb (2000) Medical Law, 3rd edition, Butterworths.

Wicks E (2001) **The right to refuse medical treatment under the European Convention on Human Rights.** *Medical Law Review,* **9,** 17.

The DVLA's At a glance guide to the current medical standards of fitness to drive can be found on their website at www.dvla.gov.uk/at_a_glance/content.htm. It is updated every six months, usually in the spring and autumn following the twice-yearly meetings of the Secretary of State's Honorary Medical Advisory Panels.

WEB-LEARNING

Medical aspects of fitness to drive

http://www.bmjlearning.com/planrecord/servlet/ResourceSearchServlet?keyWord=
epilepsyandresourceId=5001061andviewResource=

Epilepsy: diagnosis

http://www.bmjlearning.com/planrecord/servlet/ResourceSearchServlet?keyWord=
epilepsyandresourceId=5001067andviewResource=

Epilepsy: an update on treatment

http://www.bmjlearning.com/planrecord/servlet/ResourceSearchServlet?keyWord=
epilepsyandresourceId=5001069andviewResource=

Epilepsy: what to do in special circumstances

http://www.bmjlearning.com/planrecord/servlet/ResourceSearchServlet?keyWord=
epilepsyandresourceId=5001070andviewResource=

Miss H is an unmarried 38 year old legal secretary. Her long-term relationship broke up 18 months ago. She asks you to refer her to the fertility unit for IVF treatment. What are the ethical issues?

This question tests the doctor's personal and professional responsibility and the conflict between doing his best for his patients versus his responsibility to distribute scarce resources fairly.

The four deontology-based principles of medical ethics can be applied to the above scenario (see the chapter on ethical frameworks).

Autonomy: people of sound mind have the right to self-determination.

Miss H is enquiring about a course of treatment that has both benefits and harms. Is she in possession of sufficient information to make an informed decision? Her GP needs to provide Miss H with information that she can understand, to facilitate her understanding of the risks, benefits and consequences of her decision. He needs to signpost her to reliable sources of information.

Miss H needs to be informed of local IVF protocols so that she can decide what she would like to do if treatment is not available on the NHS. *Good medical practice* (GMC) advises that doctors should make their patients their first concern, and that their personal beliefs should not prejudice their patients' care.

The doctor's personal views on marriage, children or single parents should not get in the way of his professional decision-making. He needs to respect Miss H's values and decisions. If he is unable to act for Miss H because of his own strong personal beliefs, he should refer Miss H to another GP whose personal views do not prevent him from acting for the patient.

Beneficence: the actions of doctors should promote what is best for their patients.

Medically, is pregnancy in Miss H's best interests? Does Miss H have any medical conditions such as epilepsy or diabetes that would make the pregnancy risky to her health, or reduce the likelihood of successful IVF treatment, or reduce her chances of having a healthy baby?

Socially, is it in the best interests of Miss H to have a baby? Has Miss H considered other options such as fostering or adoption? Is Miss H's decision in keeping with her cultural beliefs; will she receive support from her family and community? Although not strictly a medical consideration, should Miss H's economic circumstances be discussed? Will she be able to provide for a baby? The scope of best interests extends beyond the medical considerations and encompasses ethical, social and moral considerations.

The Human Fertilisation and Embryology Authority (HFEA), which licenses and regulates IVF centres, states that a child's welfare includes the need for a father. So far this has prevented homosexual couples from seeking treatment, but changing attitudes have made it possible for unmarried couples and single women to successfully obtain treatment.

Non-maleficence: first do no harm.

Pregnancies in older woman may carry a higher risk, but older women contemplating fertility treatment may be prepared to accept the higher risk. Fertility treatment is known to be stressful, and a single mother may be less well supported and therefore more vulnerable. Depressive symptoms are more common in women after failed cycles.

Justice: Doctors must try to distribute limited resources (time, money, expensive treatments) fairly, trying to do the greatest good for the greatest number. IVF is expensive.

Local IVF guidelines try to take into account the local budget, demand for IVF treatment and demands for other forms of medical treatment.

UK practice is governed by the Human Fertilisation and Embryology Act of 1990. NICE and the HFEA consider the ethical, economic and social debate and advise on circumstances when IVF is not recommended (as in homosexual couples) but these guidelines change with changing attitudes.

VIRTUE ETHICS

A principled GP would respect his patient's autonomy and adhere to strict confidentiality. He would also be considerate of the welfare of others including the unborn child and the wider community.

LEARNING POINTS

- The four deontology-based principles of medical ethics
- Virtue ethics
- GMC: doctors should make patients their first concern
- The Human Fertilisation and Embryology Authority (HFEA)

If the examiners want to push you further, they will ask you:

- to recognise the ethical dilemma (the conflict between your role as the patient's advocate versus your gatekeeper role in the publicly funded NHS).
- to consider your options – the different ways in which you could react to the patient's request.
- What are the advantages and disadvantages of each course of action?
- Which option would you choose and why?
- What are the possible implications of your choice?
- In six months, how will you know if you had made the right choice?

RELEVANT LITERATURE

Re *Airedale NHS Trust* v. *Bland* (1993) AC 789.

Lewens T (2004) **What is genethics?** *Journal of Medical Ethics*, **30**(3), 326–328.
Genethics is the study of the ethical issues that arise out of the science of genetics and the uses of genetic technologies.

http://bmj.bmjjournals.com/cgi/collection/informed_consent

From the King's Fund: Values, voice and health: involving the public in moral decisions
http://www.kingsfund.org.uk/pdf/voices.PDF

Gifts from patients:
A patient gives you a gift. What do you do?
(The question varies from a gift of a house to a cabbage!)

This question tests the doctor's professional values and his personal responsibility. Doctors vary in their response and there is no wrong answer. However, it is advisable to have a position that is defensible.

THOUGHTS THAT MAY BE PROMPTED IN THE DOCTOR WHEN THE GIFT IS GIVEN

- A feeling of being valued and appreciated – you may have been particularly kind beyond your contractual obligations (for example, in a family bereavement), or it may make a nice change to be thanked by patients when things go right rather than only hear about complaints when things go awry.
- Embarrassed – you would find such a gift difficult to accept and to explain to your colleagues and family. What would the patient's family think and will this alter your relationship with them?
- Vague unease – you may feel that you are being bribed by the patient to provide a higher level of service or commitment. Is there a hidden agenda?
- Conflicting feelings – you may not want to offend the patient but you feel that the gift is unnecessary.

ACTIONS BY THE DOCTOR

The doctor can either accept or decline the gift.

Accept
If you think the acceptance either improves or does no harm to your relationship with the patient and his family, accept the gift.

- You need to consider the impact of accepting the gift on the wider family – your relationship with them may be adversely affected by their feelings of suspicion.
- Does your practice have a policy of sharing the gifts? Do you feel that the gift is an expression of gratitude to the team effort and is therefore best shared? Does the practice write a letter of thanks to the patient acknowledging their receipt of the gift? A business-like letter may keep the relationship from straying beyond professional boundaries.
- From a GMC probity point of view, you may want to log this into your PDP. All gifts of more than £25 should be declared and gifts of more than £100 should be registered (Health and Social Care Bill, 2001).

Decline
It seems fair to state your reasons for declining the gift to the patient.

- The refusal may be based entirely on your emotional response (that is, you are too embarrassed or uneasy, or feel the gift is disproportional to the care given).
- The refusal may be based on practice policy.
- The refusal may be on ethical grounds – is the patient competent? At the risk of sounding patronising, should you consider whether the patient or his family can afford this gift?

You suggest an **alternative** expression of thanks: You may suggest that instead of a personal gift, you would prefer a donation to the practice fund which buys new equipment for the practice, or a donation to a charity.

LEARNING POINTS

- Health and Social Care Bill, 2001
- Practice policy regarding gifts
- GMC probity

In answering this question, it is important to recognise:

- the possible effects of accepting or rejecting the gift,
- the pros and cons of each course of action and
- the implication of the action on your relationships with the patient, the family and members of the PHCT

ADDITIONAL INFORMATION

Lillis S (2004) What is good general practice?: three different views. *New Zealand Family Physician*, **31**(2), 78–83. http://www.rnzcgp.org.nz/NZFP/Issues/April2004/Lillis_Apr04.pdf

This qualitative study explored the differences in values and beliefs concerning quality in primary health care among three groups of people: patients, general practitioners and an organisation responsible for public funding of general practice services. The study found conflicting values among the three groups. Differences in the definition of quality in primary health care were pivotal in understanding why such conflicts occur.

- Public health funders maintain a population focus.
- Patients and general practitioners value the relational aspect of medicine.
- Patients believe there should be a greater emphasis on the service component of the interaction, but that trust and care comprise part of the ideal attributes of a doctor/patient relationship.

'Should doctors ever deceive their patients?' See: www.medicalethicist.net, which gives information on research into the above question (click 'research').

RELEVANT LITERATURE

GMC. **Good medical practice:** http://www.gmc-uk.org/standards/good.htm
Read http://careerfocus.bmjjournals.com/cgi/content/full/327/7417/s100:
Kirkpatrick A (2003) **Dealing with amorous advances from patients.** *BMJ,* **327,**
    7417, s100.

This question deals with personal growth in the context of working with colleagues.

A stressed partner could be recognised by the following features:

Emotion: The emotional response to simple queries provokes disproportional anger, irritation and apathy. The person appears tired, cynical and expresses feelings of low self-esteem.

Productivity: Productivity decreases: late for meetings / surgery, deadlines are not met; letters are not dictated; increased errors may occur; and poor decisions are made (inefficiency). Patients may complain. Other members of the PHCT may remark upon his short temper, and a fall in his standards of work.

Sickness: The partner may take time off work (repetitive absences). You may suspect alcohol or drug misuse.

DEFINE BURNOUT

Burnout is the end-stage of excessive stress. The stress can be intense, prolonged, or both. As the stress increases, productivity increases until it peaks. Beyond this, further loading on the individual leads to decreased performance (bell-shaped curve).

It is characterised by four stages: overwork, frustration, resentment and depression.

Christina Maslach, an American psychologist, drew up a scoring system to screen for burnout. She looked for features of:

- fatigue,
- depersonalisation (withdrawal from relationships; seeing people as problems / tasks) and
- reduced levels of achievement.

What factors may contribute to burnout?

Intrinsic factors
A competitive, type A personality who is driven to constantly maintain high personal standards and may be reluctant to delegate work to others for fear of failure. Lack of external interests (few hobbies).

Extrinsic factors
High patient expectation coupled with increasing litigation and patient complaints (increasing consumerism).

Politically enforced changes: isolated (single-handed) practice, especially in areas where there are difficulties in recruiting and retaining doctors (inner city); demands of the new contract; high rate of change in the way doctors work, e.g. being inspected for Q and O points by the PCT, which may be perceived as a loss of autonomy. Conflict within the practice. Long working hours, including out of hours cover; lack of variety and little challenge (GPwSIs and those with diplomas and the MRCGP are less likely to suffer burnout).

Personal factors: disenchantment with career; competing demands from family; difficulty maintaining a work/home balance.

What measures would you take to prevent burnout?

Maintain a good work/home balance.

Work: a varied work environment; good relationships, delegation; prioritisation; support network (young principals' group; Balint group; mentors). Work smart, not hard!

Home: regular holidays; sport; hobbies; friends.

LEARNING POINTS

- Maslach inventory
- Depersonalisation
- Young principals' group; Balint group

If the examiner wants to push you further, he will ask you:

- how you recognise that a colleague is stressed?
- to discuss the different ways in which doctors can reduce work stress and burnout?
- Which method(s) will you choose and why?

ADDITIONAL INFORMATION

Graske J (2003) Improving the mental health of doctors. *BMJ Career Focus*, **327**: s188.

This article states that the prevalence of any common mental disorder in doctors is thought to be as high as 28%, compared with 15% in the general population. However, two good studies (Cunningham GM, 1994) have shown mental illness in doctors to be no greater than in the general public and less than in the legal profession. Graske (2003) writes:

- Depression occurs in 10% of doctors, compared with 5% of the general population.
- Suicide rates are higher too, with male doctors twice as likely and female doctors three to four times more likely to commit suicide than the general population.
- The magnitude of addiction among medical professionals is largely unknown, but has been estimated at 1 in 15 doctors (BMA, 1998).

Certain personality types and learning styles are more susceptible to psychological difficulties in medicine. Common personality traits include perfectionism, high self-criticism, low flexibility, high discipline, idealism, and high empathy. When these traits are combined with over-commitment, social isolation, and poor coping strategies, mental distress often results.

Support services are emerging within and outside the NHS, such as the Doctors' Support Line and the National Counselling Service for Sick Doctors. Some trusts have implemented mentoring and peer support, and some medical students are receiving education regarding their own behaviour and health.

Stanton J and Caan W (2003) How many doctors are sick? *BMJ Career Focus*, **326**(7391), S97a. This paper attempted to answer the above question by:

Searching the literature: One study (Newbury-Birch *et al.*, 2002) showed that 10% of all house officers were currently depressed.

Reviewing GMC data: Of the 201 doctors under GMC supervision at 31 December 2000, 199 were for alcohol-, drug-, and mental health-related problems (GMC, March 2002).

Analysing data from the BMA counselling service: Calls taken between January 2001 and January 2002 were analysed. Approximately 35% of the health-related calls were about depression and stress.

RELEVANT LITERATURE

British Medical Association (1998) **The misuse of alcohol and other drugs by doctors.** BMA, London.

Cunningham GM (1994) **A treatment programme for physicians impaired by alcohol and other drugs.** Annals of the Royal College of Physicians and Surgeons of Canada, **27,** 219–221.

Department of Health. (2001) **Improving working lives for doctors.** London: DoH. www.doh.gov.uk/iwl

Edwards N, Kornacki M, Silversin J (2002) **Unhappy doctors: what are the causes and what can be done?** BMJ, **324,** 835–838.

Jain A, Ogden J (1999) **General practitioners' experiences of patients' complaints.** BMJ http://www.bmj.com/cgi/content/full/318/7198/1596

Miller L (2002) **Helping troubled doctors.** BMJ, **324** (suppl), S148.

Newbury-Birch D, Lowry RJ, Kamali F (2002) **The changing patterns of drinking, illicit drug use, stress, anxiety and depression in dental students in a UK dental school: a longitudinal study.** Br Dent J, **192,** 646–649.

Pattani A, Constantinovici N, Williams S (2001) **Who retires early from the NHS because of ill health and what does it cost? A national cross sectional study.** BMJ, **322,** 208–209.

Smith R (2001) **Why are doctors so unhappy?** BMJ, **322,** 1073–1074.

BMJ Careers **chronic illness matching scheme:** www.bmjcareers.com/chill/

Career focus **theme issue on doctors' wellbeing:** http://bmj.com/content/vol326/issue7391/#CAREER

The GMC publications **Supporting doctors and protecting patients** and **Good medical practice** prioritise the safety of patients.

The initiative Improving Working Lives (IWL) aims to make the workplace a healthier and more supportive place to work.

Doctors' Support Line: tel. 0870 765 0001; www.doctorsupport.org

Medical Council on Alcohol (Tel 020 7487 4445; www.medicouncilalcol.demon.co.uk)

National Counselling Service for Sick Doctors (tel. 0870 241 0535; www.ncssd.org.uk)

Sick Doctors' Trust (addicted physicians' programme) (tel 01252 345 163).

Partner smelling of alcohol:

Your senior partner comes to work for the second time smelling of alcohol. What is your response?

This question tests the doctor's professional values in the context of working with colleagues.

He needs to consider the partner, the practice, the patients and his professional obligations. One doctor in 15 is dependent on alcohol or other drugs (BMA, 1998).

Your emotional response may include:

Uneasiness

You realise that this is a serious situation and your partnership needs to take action. Tackling the problem is recommended by the GMC – doctors have a professional and ethical obligation to do no harm to their patients and to intervene when concerns for the safety of their patients arise. However, taking action will result in an emotional and financial upheaval for the practice and its patients. Some partnerships try to avoid the turbulence such a confrontation will create by denying that a problem exists – turning a blind eye amounts to collusion at the patients' expense.

Relief

You have suspected a problem exists and now you have evidence. Have suspicions been raised by colleagues or patients in the past?

Sympathy

You may be aware of the partner's problems and feel that his drinking is symptomatic of his sadness, possible depression, and burnout. You may feel that confrontation and recognition of the problem will lead to treatment of the senior partner, thus improving his long-term health.

Your actions:

Confront partner alone: less threatening to the partner but you may be intimidated by him. You may get him to admit that a problem (like depression) exists and encourage him to seek help from his GP, the Sick Doctors' Association, the BMA counselling services or the local Occupational Medicine consultant. It would be wrong for either of you to start treating the problem – the aim here is to recognise its existence and assemble a plan of action.

Discuss with other partners and/or practice manager: This encourages corporate ownership of a difficult issue and you may feel less isolated. If all of you are in agreement about the best course of action, then there will be less tension within the practice. If you are not in agreement, then you have to weigh up whether you want to 'whistleblow' while others want to 'collude', remembering that the patients' safety is paramount. It would be advisable to consult your medical defence union for advice.

Whistleblowing (McGuire, 2004): If the partner refuses to admit the problem, but you (and the partnership) disagree, then a more direct course of action is needed.

You may contact the local PCT advisor and ultimately the GMC. The aim of the GMC is to 'help doctors and protect patients'. The stated intention is not to be punitive towards underperforming doctors, but to assist them in dealing with the problems. The GMC asks two doctors (usually psychiatrists) to examine the 'sick doctor'. Their report advises on treatment and/or limitations to their medical work (such as, supervised work only, limited registration, or removal from the medical list). These limitations are removed on recovery.

Practice changes: If there are concerns about the senior partner's standard of work, then his work will need auditing, creating more work for an already strained partnership. The partnership and PCT need to discuss the financial implications of having a partner off on long-term sick leave or working within limitations. The staff morale may be adversely affected by the higher work load and the emotional burden. The partner may have difficulty reintegrating into the practice and fielding questions from colleagues and patients.

LEARNING POINTS

- It is your professional duty to recognise a problem exists
- Treating the sick doctor is not your responsibility – this is for his GP and/or psychiatrist
- Occupational medicine advice for GPs
- Whistleblowing versus collusion
- The GMC health procedures: fitness to practice; limitations to sick doctor's scope of work; and a treatment plan for the sick doctor

If the examiners want to push you further, they will question you on:

- The pros and cons of tackling the problem
- Whether you will tackle the problem yourself, or within the practice, or get external involvement
- The possible effects of either course of action on the parties concerned.

ADDITIONAL INFORMATION

Problem doctors

The GMC will investigate 'problem doctors' that are referred to them if:

- a doctor has been convicted of a criminal offence;
- there is evidence of serious professional misconduct;
- there is evidence that a doctor is not fit to practice; or
- there is evidence of 'seriously deficient performance'.

Health

The health procedures allow the GMC to act if a doctor is trying to practise despite being seriously affected by ill health. The main aim is to protect patients.

However, the GMC also encourages the sick doctor to seek treatment with a view to returning to work if possible. The most serious cases are referred to the Health Committee which can suspend or place conditions on the doctor's registration.

Conduct

The GMC conduct procedures allow the GMC to investigate allegations of serious professional misconduct, and to deal with doctors convicted of criminal offences. If a doctor is found guilty of serious professional misconduct or has been convicted of a criminal offence, the Professional Conduct Committee (PCC) may cancel, suspend or place conditions on their registration. Or they may give the doctor a warning.

Performance

The performance procedures allow the GMC to investigate doctors whose performance appears to be 'seriously deficient'. If necessary, the Committee on Professional Performance (CPP) will suspend or place conditions on the doctor's registration. After two years, registration may be suspended indefinitely.

If the GMC receives a report of poor performance, they will decide whether there is a case to answer. If there is, the GMC will send a team of trained assessors to assess the doctor's performance. The assessment will cover the doctor's:

- attitudes;
- knowledge;
- clinical and communication skills; and
- clinical records and audit results.

The assessment team will normally include two doctors from the relevant specialty and a member of the public. After the assessment, the team will report to the case co-ordinator – a medical member of the council who supervises performance cases. The case co-ordinator will decide on the next step. This may be:

- to take no further action – if the assessment has revealed no serious performance problems;
- to insist that the doctor takes action to improve his performance – if problems have been identified but the public are not at immediate risk; or
- to refer the doctor to the CPP – if serious problems have been identified and the doctor's registration needs reviewing for public safety.

McGuire R (2004) Blowing the whistle – safely. *BMJ Career Focus*, **328**, s7.

The definition of a whistleblower is somebody who exposes misconduct or malpractice within an organisation. A recent survey of NHS staff found that the culture within the NHS is improving. Of staff who had concerns about patient safety, 90% 'blew the whistle' and two thirds of them reported that they suffered no reprisals as a result and that their concerns were addressed reasonably.

The Public Interest Disclosure Act reduces the fear that staff previously felt about losing their jobs or being victimised in other ways because of raising concerns at work. The act is designed 'to promote responsible whistleblowing' while at the same time protecting individuals who make disclosures of misconduct or malpractice, or both. However, the act is not designed to protect individuals who have a personal grievance against their employers.

The charity Public Concern at Work strongly encourages all organisations to actively promote a whistleblowing policy for the protection of both the organisation and employees. Public Concern at Work has recently produced a user-friendly policy which gives useful background information on public disclosure legislation and also includes templates for letters, posters, checklists, and other documents that can be disseminated and used by employers.

RELEVANT LITERATURE

Fowlie DG (1999) **The misuse of alcohol and other drugs by doctors: a UK report and one region's response.** *Alcohol and Alcoholism*, **34**(5), 666–671. http://alcalc.oupjournals.org/cgi/content/full/34/5/666

Southgate L (2001) **The General Medical Council's Performance Procedures: the development and implementation of tests of competence with examples from general practice.** *Medical Education*, **35** (Suppl. 1), 20–28.

The GMC's fitness to practice procedures: http://www.gmc-uk.org/probdocs/default.htm and http://www.gmc-uk.org/standards/default.htm

The practice manager (PM) is late for work on most mornings. How could you, as the partner overseeing human resources, deal with this?

This question tests the doctor's communication skills in the context of working with colleagues – his management of underperforming staff.

ESTABLISH THE FACTS

Confirm your findings from a variety of sources – receptionists, practice nurses. Get details – you need to be specific about actual dates.

Is the partnership worried about general under-performance? Is the lack of punctuality a sign of slipping standards in other aspects of her work? Audit her work activities. If the concern is only about punctuality, this is a less serious issue than general under-performance.

Discuss the facts with the partners and decide what outcomes you would like as a partnership. Also decide the best time in which to have the discussion – if the concern is minor (punctuality) then perhaps the issue can be raised at the next staff performance review. However, if the concerns are greater, a meeting needs to be convened more urgently. The partnership may want to check the terms of the practice manager's contract prior to the meeting and get employment law advice. Consult the PCT or the MDU to ascertain information on the correct disciplinary proceedings. The practice manager, if in dispute with the partnership, may appear before an Employment Tribunal and the proceedings will be scrutinised.

MEETING WITH THE PRACTICE MANAGER

Assuming this is a minor issue about punctuality, it can be raised informally over coffee. 'I have noticed that you have been late on a few mornings – is everything OK?' The aim of this non-confrontational approach is to establish the reasons behind the uncharacteristic behaviour and to negotiate a win-win solution. It may be that the PM is having a minor personal problem (e.g. difficulty with the school run) and felt too embarrassed to speak to the partners about it.

The issue can also be raised at the performance review. It is important to understand the difference between a performance review (management tool) and an appraisal (educational tool).

An appraisal is a formative experience designed to facilitate the appraisee's development. It is not limited to doctors and is increasingly available to the whole PHCT. However, an appraisal is based on the agenda set by the individual and is determined by information the appraisee brings. An appraiser (the GP) cannot introduce information from outside sources at this discussion. It would be wrong to bring up a disciplinary issue at an appraisal.

PERFORMANCE REVIEW

A performance review is a discussion to assess whether an individual has satisfied the contractual requirements of the job. The employer and employee, using the employee's terms of reference, draw up a set of SMART objectives (specific, measurable, achievable, realistic, timely). At the end of the review cycle, they decide (based on the evidence) whether these objectives have been met. Punctuality is important because the practice manager needs to be at work to complete her duties and she also needs to set an example to those who fall under her line management. At the next review cycle, the practice manager needs to demonstrate that she has successfully dealt with the issue.

DISCIPLINARY MATTERS

The practice manager's contract should have included a statement about

- her rights to time off (paid and unpaid); and
- disciplinary procedures (usually in the section on notice, grievance and disciplinary procedures)

The partnership should follow these procedures – it will hold them in good stead should any disputes arise before an employment tribunal.

Half of all partnerships do not provide employees with a contract! Even fewer have systems for staff appraisal and performance reviews.

LEARNING POINTS

- Practice disciplinary procedures and employment law
- Appraisal versus performance review
- SMART objectives

If the examiner wants to push you further, he will ask you:

- to name the different ways in which a doctor can deal with underperforming staff.
- What are the possible advantages and disadvantages of each of these methods?
- Which method(s) will you choose and why?
- On reviewing your work in six months, how would you know if you had dealt with the underperforming staff member correctly?

ADDITIONAL NOTES

The role of the practice manager

Prior to 1990, practices were not reimbursed the salaries of practice managers so practices with managers disguised them as receptionists or secretaries. Annex C of the 2004 contract defines the role of practice managers and maps out three levels of competency and nine areas of responsibility.

The three levels of competency are categorised as

- administrative
- managerial
- strategic

The nine levels of responsibility are

- operation and development,
- risk management,
- partnership issues,
- patient and community services,
- finance,
- human resources,
- premises and equipment,
- information management and technology, and
- population care.

SMART objectives
- Specific: start with an active verb e.g. arrange, complete, determine, evaluate.
- Measurable: Mention should be made of quality, quantity, time and cost.
- Achievable: this should be within cost, capability and capacity parameters.
- Relevant/ Realistic: this should be relevant and realistic to the changing needs of the practice.
- Timely: Deadlines and time-frames must be identified.

Performance review cycle
- The line manager and job holder agree the job holder's objectives for the next twelve months. These objectives should be SMART, and should state when the objectives will be completed and to what standards, with an illustration of what the end product will look like.
- The line manager and job holder meet at mid-year to discuss progress against the performance agreement.
- The line manager and job holder meet at the end of the year to assess the job holder's performance. The line manager gives the job holder feedback (see section on feedback).

ADDITIONAL INFORMATION

McGuire R (2004) Grievance and discipline procedures at work. *BMJ Career Focus*, **329**(7474), 193–193. If an employer is contemplating dismissal, or loss of pay or seniority, they must follow a three-step procedure which involves:

Step 1 – Written notification

Employers must provide an employee with written information on the details about the problem that has led to dismissal or disciplinary action being considered. The employee should be invited to attend a meeting where the problem can be discussed.

Step 2 – Meeting

Both employer and employee must take reasonable steps to attend the meeting that will enable the two parties to discuss the problem. The law gives the employee the right to be accompanied at a hearing and employees should be made aware of this. Employers also need to ensure that the meeting is held in a place that is accessible by the employee and/or the person they elect to accompany them to the hearing.

The main objective of the meeting should be resolution. If the meeting is genuinely about resolution then the employer can only make a decision about how to proceed with the complaint against the employee *after* rather than during the meeting. Attempting to make a decision during the meeting is counterproductive to the process of making an informed and balanced judgement. After the meeting, the employer should inform the employee of the decision and also of their right to appeal against the decision.

Step 3 – Appeal

A further meeting should be held, if requested, in which an appeal against a decision can be made. An appeal meeting should be chaired by a more senior manager then the individual who chaired the original meeting and made the original decision. The decision from the appeal must be communicated to the employee.

If an employer does not follow the minimum procedure then an employment tribunal may judge the dismissal 'automatically unfair'.

RELEVANT LITERATURE

Stone W (2004) **Fraud in the GP surgery.** BMJ Career Focus, **329**(7467), 115–115.

The new GMS contract 2003, annex C, Competency Framework for Practice Management.

For further information on employment law, see the ACAS or the Department for Trade and Industry (dti) website. http://www.acas.org.uk/rights/discipline.html

How to communicate better with patients and colleagues http://www.bmjlearning.com/planrecord/servlet/ResourceSearchServlet?keyWord=Read%2C+reflect%2C+respond&resourceId=5003160&viewResource=

Managing complaints

A patient sees you for a repeat prescription of anti-depressants which she says were started by the senior partner one month ago. There is no record of the consultation or the medication on her computer records. You advise her that you will be happy to prescribe if she brings in her current medication. She says that she considers it poor practice that her notes are incomplete – she would like to make a complaint. Discuss the practice complaints procedure and the ways in which the practice can learn from complaints.

This question tests the doctor's communication skills in the context of caring for patients and working with colleagues.

THE COMPLAINTS PROCEDURE

Stage 1 (in-house procedures)

Complaint
↓
Complaints administrator
GP acknowledgement in 2 days
↓
Full response in 10 working days → Complainant satisfied → Yes → End

↓

Stage 2 (handled by PCT complaints manager)

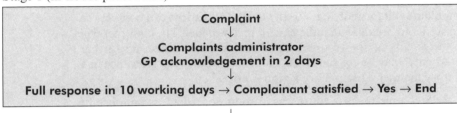

No
↓
Health authority assistance and/or conciliator
↓
Complainant satisfied → Yes → End

↓

Stage 3 (independent review panel consisting of doctors, lay people and PCT representative)

↓

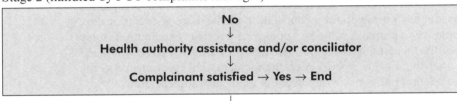

No
↓
Is an independent review panel needed?

↓

Stage 4 (the ombudsman)

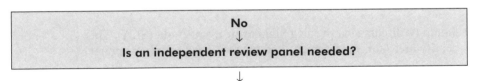

Complainant satisfied → Yes → End
No
↓
Ombudsman (answerable to Parliament)

The practice complaints procedure should be readily available in writing – usually in the practice information leaflet. It must include:

- How the complaint will be dealt with
- The purpose of the procedure
- An anticipated time-table – the practice should acknowledge receipt of the complaint within 2 days in writing. The practice should discuss the issues and respond to the complaint within 10 days. A complaint should be made within six months of the incident.
- Assurance of confidentiality
- Possible outcomes of the procedures:
  - Resolution – a meeting between the complainant and practitioner is held only if both parties genuinely want this and the meeting has a clear purpose.
  - If the issue remains unresolved, the PCT manager can act as an in-house intermediary. The conciliators do not report details of the case to the PCT. Their job is to facilitate discussion.
  - The complaint will formally pass to the PCT. The patient can contact the PCT convener to organise an independent review panel. The convener will review the details of the complaint and may decide to take no further action. A panel may be convened – the aim is to resolve the grievance in a conciliatory manner. Disciplinary action is not taken.

In 1996 a new NHS complaints procedure was introduced. It had two important aims:

- It separated complaints from disciplinary procedures. The new complaints procedure sought to bring about a conciliation of the damaged relationship. Most people who complain want an apology and a clear explanation in lay language of the incident, with reassurance that preventative action will taken to ensure that there is no repetition of the incident. This is contrary to the popular belief that patients are only seeking financial compensation.
- Complaints should be dealt with informally and locally. In 1996, more than 90% of complaints were dismissed or resolved.

HOW CAN THE PRACTICE LEARN FROM THE COMPLAINT?

The complaint should be discussed at the next Significant Event Audit (SEA). The PHCT should identify areas for improvement and take actions to prevent similar occurrences.

The doctor should reflect on the incident and note it in his PDP for discussion at his appraisal.

LEARNING POINTS

- The 4 stage complaints procedure
- Possible outcomes: resolution, conciliators, pass to the PCT
- Complaints are separated from disciplinary procedures
- Learn from complaints – SEAs

ADDITIONAL INFORMATION

Avoiding complaints

Pre-empt a complaint. If the doctor recognises that he has had a dysfunctional consultation, a quick phone call may head off a complaint.

If a doctor makes an incorrect or delayed diagnosis, the GMC advises that a full and honest explanation with an apology should be provided.

Good communication reduces complaints (Beckman *et al.*, 1994).

Common complaints (1998 data from County Durham)

- The patient disliked the attitude of the GP and there was a breakdown in communication (including failure to visit or refer) – 30%
- Delayed or incorrect diagnoses – 28%
- Complaints about staff or the premises – 21%
- Problems with the practice management – 18%
- Others (including removal from list) – 3%

Why complaints are stressful to doctors

Doctors feel that patients who complain have power over them, making them feel helpless and uncertain.

Doctors feel that they are working hard for people who have very high expectations, are not particularly grateful and very quick to blame them for anything that goes wrong with their care. Doctors feel devalued by the increasing consumerism of patients and very rarely separate complaints from litigation in their thoughts.

Complaints and child protection

In 2004, the Royal College of Paediatrics and Child Health (RCPCH) completed part one of a two-phase survey into complaints made against paediatricians. Since 1993, there has been more than a five-fold increase in the number of complaints made to the RCPCH. The RCPCH feel that these complaints and the accompanying high profile reports to the media make doctors involved in child protection feel undervalued and unprotected.

The president of the RCPCH, Alan Craft, thinks that there are many reasons why complaints have increased:

1. There is now a general complaining culture in society.
2. It is a natural reaction for parents who have been accused of harming their children to find some way of hitting back.

3. There has been an orchestrated campaign against certain specialists, by a small group of parents, mostly using the internet.

However, if paediatricians are reluctant to report child abuse cases, then children will be unprotected.

From: www.mps.org.uk

The Shipman Inquiry's 5th report, due in late 2004, is likely to address complaints handling in some detail. New complaints regulations will be issued in 2005, once the DoH has given the Shipman recommendations, together with those from the Ayling, Neale, Kerr and Haslam Inquiries, proper consideration.

Guidance to support implementation of the National Health Service (Complaints) Regulations 2004 can be found on the DoH website, www.dh.gov.uk.

Baker R (2004) Patient-centred care after Shipman. *Journal of the Royal Society of Medicine*, **97**(4), 161–165.

The Shipman case has implications beyond adjustment to a limited number of systems. Although reform of some systems is required, including certification, monitoring and complaints, doctors must also confront the deeper issues that allowed these systems to deteriorate and Shipman, the murderer, to prosper. The key issue is how doctors think about themselves in relation to their patients. The main task for the profession and its organisations is a process of renewal whereby the interests of patients genuinely come first.

Why patients sue their doctors (from www.mps.org.uk):

- More than 50% of 263 patients who sued their doctor claimed that they were so turned off by the doctor that they wanted to sue him/her before the alleged event occurred. (Mangels, 1991)
- Negative communication behaviour by doctors increases litigious intent – even when there have been no adverse outcomes. (Lester and Smith, 1993)
- 71% of litigation is related to a poor relationship / communication between doctor and patient, with four main reasons for criticising the clinician:
  - deserting the patient
  - devaluing the patient and/or family views
  - poor delivery of information
  - failing to understand patient's point of view (Beckman *et al.*, 1994).

RELEVANT LITERATURE

Beckman HB, Markakis KM, Suchman AL, Frankel RM (1994) The doctor–patient relationship and malpractice: lessons from plaintiff depositions. *Arch. Int. Med.*, **154** (June), 1365–1370.

Lester GW and Smith SG (1993) Listening and talking to patients: a remedy for malpractice suits? *West. J. Med.* see http://www.medicalprotection.org/medical/united_kingdom/publications/casebook/2004_4_care_ref.aspx

Mangels LS (1991) Tips from doctors who've never been sued. *Med. Econ.*, **68**(4), 56–8, 60–4.

This question tests the doctor's communication skills and professional values in the context of caring for the patient.

The removal of a patient from the practice list can be a difficult and upsetting experience for both the patient and the doctor. Removal usually occurs when the doctor–patient relationship has irreparably broken down, as is likely to be the case in the above scenario. Occasionally the breakdown occurs with one doctor rather than the practice, and another partner may agree to take the patient on.

The Patients' Liaison Group of the RCGP has prepared guidance on the removal procedures. The guidance states reasons when it is justifiable for practices to remove patients and also highlights areas when it would be unreasonable for doctors to remove patients.

JUSTIFIABLE REASONS FOR REMOVAL

- Violence, by the patient, their family members or their unchained pets
  - towards any member of the PHCT (in surgery or when visited)
  - towards other patients in the practice
  - towards practice property – physical damage
  - the violence may be physical or verbal (including racial abuse)
- Crime and deception
  - steals from the practice (therefore the theft of the laptop is grounds for removal)
  - fraudulently obtains drugs for non-medical reasons
  - gives false information to obtain benefits
- Distance
  - when the patient moves out of the practice and fails to register with a new GP

UNJUSTIFIABLE REASONS FOR REMOVAL

- Simply because the care of the patient is costly or time-consuming (very disabled; very demanding)
- You cannot discriminate against a patient on grounds of age, gender, ethnic origin, religious belief or sexual orientation
- Refusal of treatment – smears, childhood immunisation, non-compliance with therapeutic advice

Grey areas (these are reasons where it is not normally justifiable to remove a patient from the list but on closer scrutiny, good reasons may exist)

- Complaints – especially if the patient persists in making unjustifiable or malicious complaints about the standards of the practice or members of the PHCT.

Patients are removed only when the practice feels that the doctor–patient relationship has irretrievably broken down. The circumstances surrounding the breakdown may be perceived differently by the doctor and the patient. Attempts should be made to restore the relationship. If a GP decides there is a need to remove a patient, the patient's family should not automatically be removed too.

How would you go about removing a patient from the list?

It is important to document in detail:

- any incidents that have led to the removal,
- any steps that have been taken to retrieve the situation,
- the specific reasons for the removal and
- the process of removing the patient.

The RCGP Patients' Liaison Group, in their guidance, advises that steps be taken with the practice, the patient, and the PCT.

Steps to be taken within the practice
- Inform all appropriate members of the practice about the problem.
- Confidentially explore possible reasons for the patient's actions (cultural differences, mental illness).
- Is the practice contributing to the deteriorating relationship (poorly performing receptionist, stressed GP)? Could these be remedied?

Steps to be taken with the patient
- Inform the patient personally. Most doctors arrange a meeting with the patient and write to the patient, but usually after seeking advice from their defence union.
- Discuss reasons for removal with the patient. A neutral third party (perhaps a member of the patient participation group) may facilitate the discussion.
- Listen to the patient's perspective and try to negotiate a solution.
- Suggest that another GP within the practice may better fit with the patient's needs and expectations.

Steps to be taken if discussions fail
- Inform the patient about other local practices with whom he may want to register.

Removal procedures
- Inform the PCT in writing.
- It is advisable to write to the patient informing him of his removal. Patients should be given a written explanation for their removal and notice of it. This is in line with GMC advice and contractual requirements (clauses 192–209 of the new General Medical Services contract or Primary Medical Services requirements.)
- There will be rare occasions when it will be inappropriate to write, such as when a practice needs to remove a patient immediately, because he has been violent to a staff member and they fear for the safety of the doctors and other staff.

- Reassure the patient that he will not be left without a GP – give him information about registering elsewhere. However, where violence has been a factor it will be the responsibility of the PCT to arrange primary care services, if necessary, within a more secure setting.
- The doctor should speak to his medical union.

LEARNING POINTS

- Guidance from RCGP Patients' Liaison Group
- Justifiable and unjustifiable reasons for removal
- Facilitated discussion
- Removal procedure – PCT, MDU

If the examiner wants to push you further, he will ask:
- In the above scenario, will you remove the patient from your list? Why?
- What are the possible advantages and disadvantages, for patients and for doctors, of removing patients from their lists?

RELEVANT LITERATURE

The Royal College of General Practitioners also has specific guidelines for GPs on removing patients from lists (Removal of patients from GPs' lists: Guidance for college members), http://www.rcgp.org.uk/corporate/position/removal_of_patients_from_gp_lists.pdf

This question tests the doctor's communication skills in the context of caring for patients as well as his personal responsibility in using limited resources effectively.

O'Dowd in 1988 used the term heartsink patients to describe patients who:

- Consult frequently
- Have features of psychosomatic illness, with underlying depression or anxiety into which they have no insight
- Invoke feelings of anger, resentment and despair in the doctor.

The patients tend to be:

- Female
- Of lower socio-economic class
- Older (over 40 years)
- and have thick medical notes (with lots of previous medical interventions and referrals).

Good (1994) says that heartsinks look at medicine as a salvation – medicine influences and suggests, or in some cases wholly supplies the character and identity of some individuals' personal suffering and is the apparent source of their salvation or redemption.

Gerrard and Riddell (1998) said that one doctor's set of heartsinks is not the same as another's, implying that the problem does not lie solely with the patient; the patient–doctor relationship is dysfunctional.

Conflict arises because the patient and doctor approach the problem from different angles. The patient is looking to medicine to improve their happiness (soteriological health beliefs). The doctor has a limited model of medicine, usually a biological, disease-focused model, and lacks an holistic approach.

Mathers *et al.* (1995) found that doctors who have heartsinks are more likely to:

- be inexperienced
- have a greater perceived workload and lower job satisfaction
- be lacking in postgraduate qualifications and communication skills

Groves (1978) defined four types of difficult patient:

1. Dependent clinger: They make repeated requests for reassurance and have an inexhaustible need for love and attention, provoking resentment in the doctor. The game they play is 'Poor me!'.
2. Entitled demander: Complains about imagined shortcomings in the service provided. They try to manipulate the doctor through the use of intimidation and provoke feelings of guilt and anxiety. This is a reflection of their own fear and insecurity. The game they play is 'I'm going to take this further!'.

3. Manipulative health rejector: They constantly return complaining that their treatment is not working. They seek attention rather than relief from their symptoms and tend to play the ' Yes, but…' game.
4. Self-destructive denier: Refuses to accept that their behaviour affects their illness, and will not modify their habits, hence self-harming to the point of destruction. These include the incurable alcoholics and non-compliant diabetics. They provoke rejection in the doctor. The game they play is 'Kick me!'.

What are your coping strategies for dealing with Mrs MB? The doctor needs to formulate an appropriate and shared plan with Mrs MB. He also needs to be aware of the feelings Mrs MB is provoking and deal with these appropriately so that the relationship does not deteriorate.

A useful management strategy was outlined by Barsky *et al.* (1999):

1. Rule out the presence of diagnosable medical disease: Review the notes. Be careful about ordering investigations and referring the patient – this fosters the sick role and negative tests usually heighten the patient's anxiety.
2. Search for psychiatric disorders: Look for depression, anxiety and panic disorders as these may present with physical symptoms.
3. Build a collaborative alliance with the patient: Acknowledge the patient's suffering but be careful not to encourage the sick role. See one doctor for regular, planned follow-up and avoid examinations unless new symptoms develop. Listening to the patient can be therapeutic for the patient – this is called 'holding' the patient's anxieties. However, recognise that these patients are manipulative and demanding, so set out boundaries such as the frequency of meetings and the 'rules of engagement'.
4. Set goals for treatment:
   a. Reduction in severity or frequency of symptoms and improvement in function – help the patient cope rather than searching for a cure.
   b. Patients should be actively involved in their management decisions – they should not assume a passive role.
   c. Realistic, incremental goals should be set, e.g. graduated exercise programmes.
5. Providing limited reassurance: Patients need to be told that lethal or progressive disease has been excluded and an exhaustive search for the root cause is not indicated. Rather, it would be more productive to concentrate on reducing symptoms – this acknowledges their symptomatology and refocuses their goals.
6. Prescribing cognitive behavioural therapy and/or antidepressants if patients do not respond to the previous five steps: CBT is shown to be effective in the treatment of medically unexplained symptoms such as IBS, fibromyalgia and chronic fatigue syndrome. CBT helps patients to find alternative explanations for their symptoms – they alter their health beliefs and change their illness behaviour. A meta-analysis involving 6500 patients showed that anti-depressants can provide useful symptomatic relief whether depression is present or not (NNT 3). Benefit is seen within 1–7 days.

The doctor's coping strategies:

1. Doctors should recognise the feelings provoked by heartsinks. Those who are more self-aware and have better consulting and counselling skills cope better.
2. Heartsinks do occur. However, the emotional burden can be reduced by:
   a. Improving the doctor's working environment – allow longer consulting by having flexible appointment lengths
   b. Discussing in peer / Balint groups
   c. Housekeeping (Neighbour) – deal honestly with the emotions invoked by the demanding patient.

LEARNING POINTS

- Heartsinks, or patients with medically unexplained symptoms (MUS), invoke resentment and despair in their doctors
- Soteriological health beliefs – looking to medicine for salvation
- Dysfunctional doctor–patient relationship
- Groves' classification of heartsinks
- Collaborative alliance with patient defining rules of engagement
- Evidence for efficacy of CBT and anti-depressants

ADDITIONAL INFORMATION

Ring A, Dowrick C *et al.* (2004) Do patients with unexplained physical symptoms pressurise general practitioners for somatic treatment?: a qualitative study. *BMJ*, **328**(7447) 1057–60.

This study looked at 7 general practices in Merseyside, England. 36 patients with medically unexplained symptoms from 21 general practices had their consultations audio-taped. The study concluded that most patients with unexplained symptoms received somatic interventions from their general practitioners but had not requested them. Though such patients apparently seek to engage the general practitioner by conveying the reality of their suffering, general practitioners respond by treating their symptoms.

Dowrick FC, Ring A *et al.* (2004) Normalisation of unexplained symptoms by general practitioners: a functional typology. *British Journal of General Practice*, **54**(500), 165–170.

This study concluded that:

- Normalisation without explanation, i.e. rudimentary reassurance and the authority of a negative test result, rendered somatic management more likely.
- Normalisation with ineffective explanation provided a tangible physical explanation for symptoms, unrelated to patients' expressed concerns. This was also counterproductive.

- Normalisation with effective explanation provided tangible mechanisms grounded in patients' concerns, often linking physical and psychological factors. These explanations were accepted by patients; those linking physical and psychological factors contributed to psychosocial management outcomes.

These findings can inform the development of well-grounded educational interventions for GPs.

Woivalin T, Krantz G *et al*. (2004) Medically unexplained symptoms: perceptions of physicians in primary health care. *Family Practice*, **21**(2), 199–203.

The aim of this Swedish study was to explore GPs' perceptions and ways of managing patients with medically unexplained symptoms (MUS). The GPs described how they used four different approaches to manage patients with MUS:

- a biomedical,
- a psychological,
- an educational and
- a psychosocial approach.

Different approaches were used, depending on the patient and the situation, and the GPs even switched approach when working with the same patient.

The study concluded that in their work with patients with MUS, GPs need support and further training to improve the way the biomedical frame of reference is integrated with the humanistic perspective.

RELEVANT LITERATURE

ABC of psychological medicine. *BMJ*, **325**, 265–268 and **325**, 323–326.

Barsky AJ, Peekna HM, and Borus JF (2001) **Somatic symptom reporting in women and men.** *J. Gen. Intern. Med*, **16**(4), 266–75.

Butler CC, Evans M *et al*. (2004) **Medically unexplained symptoms: the biopsychosocial model found wanting.** *Journal of the Royal Society of Medicine*, **97**(5), 219–22.

Campion-Smith C (2004) **Surviving and thriving with difficult and demanding patients.** *BMJ Career Focus*, **329,** 197–198.

Drugs and Therapeutics Bulletin Vol 39 No1 p5.

Gerrard TJ and Riddell JD (1998) **Difficult patients: black holes and secrets.** *BMJ*, **297**, 1295–8.

Good BJ (1994) Medicine, rationality and experience: an anthropological perspective. Cambridge University Press, New York.

Groves JE (1978) **Taking care of the hateful patient.** *New England Journal of Medicine*, **298**, 883–7.

Mathers N, Jones N, and Hannay D (1995) **Heartsink patients: a study of their general practitioners.** *Br J Gen Pract*, **45**(395), 293–6.

O'Dowd TC (1988) **Five years of heartsink patients in general practice.** *BMJ*, **297,** 528–530.

The Bath VTS website provides a comprehensive summary on patients with medically unexplained symptoms and has an excellent survival guide on how to deal with heartsinks. See:
http://www.mharris.eurobell.co.uk/newgpr/spring03/heartsin.htm

This question tests the doctor's professional values.

The ethical dilemma is the doctor's conflict between his responsibility to act in his patient's best interests as well as a professional duty to validate sickness, thus acting as social security policeman.

ETHICAL THEORIES

Doctors are most familiar with the four ethical principles of autonomy, beneficence (doing good), non-maleficence (not doing harm) and justice. However, there are three more ethical theories that can be applied to the above scenario:

- **Duty-based ethics** (deontology) – These state that an action is right if it is in accord with a moral rule or principle. Certain acts are wrong in themselves, independent of their foreseeable consequences.

   With regard to the above scenario, lying is wrong, so the doctor should not testify in a written statement that the patient was ill three days ago. He would be able to say that the patient tells him that she was ill three days ago, but not having seen or examined her during her illness, he cannot objectively make this statement (a private note or a Med 3).

   However, beneficence (doing good) and non-maleficence (not doing harm) also need to be considered. The doctor would be doing the best for his patient (acting beneficently) if he issued a note to help her with the difficulties she is having with her demanding employer. After all, the patient has done nothing wrong. She knew that she had a minor ailment and took responsibility for her own health – her health-seeking behaviour was entirely appropriate. However, her employer's attitude is encouraging doctor-dependence and inappropriate presentations to an already overstretched health service. If the doctor refuses to provide a note, he is taking appropriate action against the employer; however, this could be harmful to his patient (against the principle of non-maleficence). He could be damaging the doctor–patient trust. If he refuses to provide a note on the grounds that he did not see her when she was ill, the patient may decide to present with minor symptoms on the next occasion – the doctor would therefore be promoting inappropriate health-seeking behaviour.

- **Utilitarianism ethics, particularly consequentialism** – This principle states that an action is right if it promotes the best consequences – the greatest good or happiness for the greatest number. Those actions that promote, or intend to promote, more happiness are better than those that promote less happiness. A weakness of this theory is that it is not possible to measure happiness.

  With regard to the scenario, if the doctor:
  1. Provides a note: the patient and the employer would be happy. The doctor would have preserved a trusting relationship with his patient and had a quick non-confrontational consultation – therefore making the doctor happy too.
  2. Does not provide a note: The NHS has a finite number of resources and stretching these resources to provide a cheap occupational health service to private companies reduces the time available for seeing and treating ill patients. The NHS and society benefit from having a tough policy on the issuing of sick notes. The long term benefit / happiness to society outweighs the short term benefit to the patient, employer and doctor.

- **Virtue ethics** – This principle states that an action is right if it is what a virtuous person would do in the circumstances. A virtuous person is someone of good moral character, i.e. he is kind, generous, and empathetic.

  With regard to the scenario, if the doctor:
  1. Provides a note: He would be acting kindly and empathetically to his patient's needs.
  2. Does not provide a note: He would be acting responsibly and rationing limited resources fairly.

A weakness of this theory is that it is tied to cultural norms – the GMC's *Good medical practice* states that it is the primary duty of doctors to make the care of their patients their first concern. Therefore in the current cultural climate, it can be argued that the autonomy of patients takes precedence over the doctors' gatekeeper role – hence a virtuous doctor would make the happiness of his patient his first concern.

THE LAW

- The law states that employees may self-certify their illness for seven days before there is any need for an official DoH sick note.
- Employers should provide a self-certification certificate (SC2) so that employees can declare their illness (strictly they do not need to do this for their first three days of illness).
- If the illness continues for more than seven days, then the employee's GP can issue an official DoH statement (called Med3) as a statement of the illness.
- FMed 3: Can be completed by a GP, a hospital doctor or an alternative practitioner, such a chiropractor, to certify periods off work lasting more than seven days. The doctor needs to have examined the patient first and the Med3 is issued within a day of that clinical contact.

- FMed 5: This form is used if:
  1. The patient requires a statement for a past period of illness during which he saw his doctor but for which no doctor's statement was issued.
  2. A doctor wishes to advise a patient, whom he has not examined, to refrain from work provided he has received an adequate written report within the last month from another doctor.

If an employee requires a 'sick note' for an illness of less than seven days' duration, then a private doctor's statement may be provided. The fee for this is £10, which is a set BMA rate, to be met either by the patient or the employer.

LEARNING POINTS

- Duty-based ethics (deontology)
- Utilitarianism ethics, particularly consequentialism
- Virtue ethics
- Self-certification certificate (SC2)
- FMed 3
- FMed 5

ADDITIONAL INFORMATION

Is the UK in danger of becoming a nanny state?

The Chancellor Gordon Brown unveiled his pre-budget report on 2 December 2004. This included the following issues with implications for primary healthcare:

- Employment advisers are to be based in GPs' surgeries in an attempt to reduce reliance on long-term incapacity benefit.
- The Government will aim to improve employer and GP awareness of the implications of sickness absence. GPs, the report said, have: 'a key role to play in ensuring that their advice supports the recovery and rehabilitation of patients and, where appropriate, encourages a return to work or work-related activity'.

The BMA's response to the Government was:

- GPs will welcome practical measures to help their patients back to work where appropriate. However, the proposed pilots for Employment Advisers in surgeries will need to demonstrate that the problems currently experienced by many practices – such as lack of staff, money and space – can be resolved.
- There can be many barriers preventing a speedy return to work including inflexibility in the workplace and inadequate occupational health advice, and these problems also have to be addressed if substantial progress is to be made.

See: http://news.bbc.co.uk/nol/shared/bsp/hi/pdfs/02_12_04_pbr04_chap04_394.pdf – accessed 04 December 2004

This question tests a doctor's professional values and personal responsibility in the context of patient care.

This question raises some important issues:

- Professional
- Medico-legal
- Ethical

PROFESSIONAL

The public has certain expectations of doctors and doctors have certain responsibilities to their patients. These are stated in the GMC's *Good medical practice:*

'You must not allow your personal relationships to undermine the trust which patients place in you. In particular, you must not use your professional position to establish or pursue a sexual or improper emotional relationship with a patient or someone close to them.'

If doctors were allowed to have relationships with their patients, they could take advantage of vulnerable people, thus abusing their position of trust.

If patients were allowed to have relationships with their doctors, they could manipulate the doctor's position of power to their own ends, i.e. ask for unnecessary prescriptions / referrals / preferential treatment.

If the doctor–patient relationship were not kept professional, both parties would lose trust in the system. Doctors would worry about being accused of behaving unethically and may practice defensively, i.e. not do intimate examinations for fear of litigation. Patients would worry about the necessity of such procedures and may refrain from telling doctors about certain symptoms. It is therefore in the public's interest that both parties trust each other.

MEDICO-LEGAL

At what stage is an examination improper? Flirting versus sex? Would revealing a latent attraction damage the relationship even more? When can you date a patient?

ETHICAL

Autonomy: If both parties may be consenting adults, and neither is taking advantage of each other, why stop true love?!

Beneficence: Are single-handed doctors in remote areas allowed to form relationships or are they supposed to lead a life of celibacy? In such a remote community, not having a doctor may be worse than having a doctor who develops a healthy adult relationship with someone in the community who by default happens to be a patient.

Non-maleficence: The doctor–patient relationship needs to be on a professional basis to protect the trust patients have in their doctors and vice versa.

Justice: If doctors could establish relationships with their patients, would they treat these patients preferentially at the public's expense? Would they spend more time with these patients, give them more expensive treatments, refer them faster?

LEARNING POINTS

- Abuse of the doctor's position of trust
- Ethical arguments

ADDITIONAL INFORMATION

The case below was published in UK Casebook, Nov 2004. See: http://www.medicalprotection.org/medical/united_kingdom/publications/casebook/2004_4_liaisons.aspx for the full case.

A recent case (*CRHP* v. *GMC* [2004] EWHC 1850 (Admin)) at the UK High Court has highlighted the severe consequences for doctors who develop sexual relationships with their patients. In this case, a senior and experienced GP had an affair with a married patient, which lasted for more than 12 months until their respective partners discovered what was going on. Eventually, the matter was brought to the attention of the General Medical Council (GMC).

Although it had never, at any time, been suggested that the relationship was non-consensual, when the matter was considered by the GMC it was reported that the patient had been in a vulnerable state; she had been consulting the doctor concerned about emotional problems, and it was alleged that he had effectively pressurised her into pursuing the relationship.

At the GMC hearing, the doctor admitted the charges against him and effectively pleaded guilty to serious professional misconduct. However, in view of his undoubted competence, and the enormous groundswell of support he received from the local population, the GMC decided not to erase or suspend him from the register. He was allowed to continue practising, subject to the condition that he worked in a supervised capacity for two years.

The Council for the Regulation of Healthcare Professionals (now known as the Council for Healthcare Regulatory Excellence or CHRE) have powers to challenge decisions made by the GMC. They took this matter to the High Court, arguing that the decision not to erase the doctor was 'unduly lenient'. The High Court agreed; it determined that, as a minimum, the GMC should have suspended the doctor from practice. The court stated that this was necessary to 'send out the right signal to the profession and to the public and to mark the seriousness of the misconduct'.

Comment

Regulators take the view that the sexual relationship between doctors and their patients can never be considered truly mutual and based on an equal footing; it would always be viewed to some extent as an abuse of the trust that the patient reposes in the doctor. The message from this case is very clear; whatever the circumstances, doctors should never enter into sexual relationships with their patients.

This question tests the doctor's communication skills in the context of working with colleagues.

Complicated questions can be answered using a simple format called the '**5 Ws** and **1 H**': what, when, why, where, who and how.

WHAT IS LEADERSHIP?

Leadership covers a broad spectrum of behaviours and requires many different personal qualities. What is common to leaders is the ability to influence. A leader uses the following behaviours to influence others, particularly he is able to:

- direct and co-ordinate the work of others,
- build, support and work with teams,
- work effectively as part of a team,
- negotiate and consult effectively.

A leader displays the following qualities:

- Charismatic – he is inspirational and empowers others
- Enthusiastic – able to enthuse others
- Democratic – he is respectful of the team's views
- Visionary – he is innovative and sees the wider view
- Organised – he uses time and resources effectively; he is able to manage conflict well.

The organisation usually defines its overarching aims, which are then broken down into particular objectives which are met by the completion of specific tasks. Leadership is needed at all of these levels. For example, the aim of a practice is to achieve the maximum number of Quality and Outcome points. The process can be visualised as detailed below:

Aim (e.g. get lots of Q and O points)
↓
Objectives (as set out in nGMS contract)
↓
Tasks needed to meet objectives (set up templates, audit)

HOW DO LEADERS LEAD?

There are several styles of leadership:

1. Authoritarian – gives clear directions for specific tasks.
2. Authoritative – states the overall objectives and delegates the tasks needed to achieve these to his team.

3. Democratic – brings together the expertise of the team members to deliver the objectives.
4. Task-orientated – completes a specific task to a high standard. The task is well-defined and the obstacles which hinder the accomplishment of the task are tackled.
5. Developmental – develops the individual team members so that the team has more skills and is capable of doing more.

WHEN IS LEADERSHIP NEEDED?

Change is constantly occurring in general practice at all levels. Leadership is needed to manage the changes effectively.

WHERE IS LEADERSHIP NEEDED?

The opportunities to demonstrate leadership are present in everyday work – with patients, within the practice team, in the PCT and in the wider community, as well as both regional and national levels.

WHY IS LEADERSHIP NEEDED?

Good leaders can drive innovation in general practice, improving the working lives of colleagues and the delivery of care to patients. Poor and ineffectual leaders can do damage to both. Leaders are the focal point of contact. They take overall responsibility and are accountable for the resources they use.

WHO MAKES A GOOD LEADER?

Depending on the circumstances, different styles of leadership are appropriate, e.g. innovative partners who built up a practice 20 years ago to provide a very good palliative care service may be reluctant to let this service be taken over by specialist palliative care nurses. They may continue to prioritise palliative care over new practice needs, such as clinical governance activity. Task-orientated or developmental leadership may now be needed.

A good leader will manage change effectively, so the person singled out from the team to lead depends on the nature of the change. The optimal team was described by Dr Meredith Belbin (1969). He said that a cohesive effective team must contain a variety of personality traits, intellectual styles and behaviours. His optimal team consisted of eight players which he called:

Type	Typical features	Positive qualities	Allowable weaknesses
Chair	Calm, self-confident, controlled	Welcoming of contributions while maintaining a strong sense of objectives	Of average intellect and creative ability
Shaper	Highly strung, out-going, dynamic	Has drive – challenges inertia and complacency	Easily irritated and impatient
Company worker	Conservative, dutiful and predictable	Well-organised and practical. Hard working and self-disciplined	Can be inflexible and unresponsive to proven ideas
Team worker	Socially orientated, rather mild and sensitive	Responds to people and promotes team spirit	Indecisive in a crisis
Plant	Individualistic, serious-minded and unorthodox	Genius, imagination, intellect, knowledge	Inclined to disregard practical details or protocols
Resource investigator	Extroverted, enthusiastic, communicative	Social networker, responds to challenge	Liable to lose interest once the initial fascination has passed
Monitor–Evaluator	Sober, unemotional, prudent	Judgemental, critical, hard-hearted	Lacks inspiration or the ability to motivate others
Completer–Finisher	Painstaking, orderly, conscientious, anxious	Follows things through, perfectionist	A tendency to worry about small things. A resistance to 'let go'

LEARNING POINTS

- Leadership is the ability to influence
- Leadership is needed at all levels (to deliver aims, objectives and tasks)
- Styles of leadership: authoritarian, democratic, task-orientated, transformational
- Belbin's optimal team consisting of eight members

ADDITIONAL INFORMATION

Definitions of leadership are varied. Recent definitions have focused on vision building and empowering others.

Kurt Lewin (cited in Iles and Sutherland, 2001) discussed participative styles of leadership. These, he believes, will lead to increased job satisfaction and higher performance.

Contingency theories argue that an effective leadership style varies according to the context. Hersey and Blanchard (cited in Iles and Sutherland, 2001) wrote about situational leadership, task behaviour and relational behaviour. Task behaviour focuses on defining roles and responsibilities whereas relational behaviour is more about providing support to teams.

Instrumental theories stress task- and person-oriented behaviour (e.g. participation, delegation) by the leader to gain effective performance from others.

Inspirational theories include charismatic and transformational leadership. The charismatic leader appeals to values and vision – he enthuses others, raises confidence and motivates the team for change. Charismatic leaders have a compelling vision that draws in commitment and acceptance of change, and offers a potential for anyone to grow and develop with the vision. They inspire trust, loyalty, devotion, commitment, inspiration, and admiration. The term transformational leadership is sometimes used instead of charismatic leadership. This offers a distinction between transformational (takes people beyond self-interest, raises motivation and moral commitment) and transactional leadership (the exchange of rewards / threats for compliance).

Informal leadership looks at behaviours associated with those who are not appointed to authority but assume leadership in other ways.

Path-goal theory looks at what leaders must do to motivate people to perform well and to get satisfaction from work.

The choice of leadership style depends on the task and the individual e.g. routine tasks = supportive style, complex = directive leadership.

Bennis (cited in Iles and Sutherland, 2001) puts forward some specific differences between management and leadership. A manager is an administrator – he maintains and controls systems. A leader innovates, develops, focuses on people and inspires trust. Bennis also distinguishes between transformational (doing the right thing) and transactional leadership (doing things right). This distinction is often quoted as the difference between management and leadership.

RELEVANT LITERATURE

Belbin M (1969) **Management teams: why they succeed or fail**. Butterworth-Heinemann.
Iles V and Sutherland K (2001) Organisational change: managing change in the NHS [online]. NHS SDO R and D Programme, London. Available from www.sdo.lshtm.ac.uk

Maccoby M (2000) **Understanding the difference between management and leadership.** *Research Technology Management*, Vol. 43, No. 1 Jan–Feb. pp. 57–59.

Senge P (1990) **The fifth discipline. The art and practice of the learning organisation.** *Doubleday/Century Business*, London.

Zand D (1995) Force field analysis, cited in Iles V and Sutherland K (2001) **Organisational change. Managing change in the NHS.** *NCCSDO*, London.

Your practice nurse team puts forward a request that one of the nurses be trained in nurse prescribing. What is your response?

This question tests the doctor's professional values in the context of working with colleagues.

Recognise:

- The face of general practice and indeed medicine is changing. The roles of nurses are developing to embrace activities such as prescribing which were traditionally done only by doctors.
- There is a need and government agenda to improve patient access to a clinician, and by counting nurses as autonomous clinicians, the government can meet waiting time targets more easily.
- However, doctors feel that their professional responsibilities are being undervalued and that their work is being passed onto nurses who have inadequate training and are cheaper to employ.

Options and implications

- Support the nurse's application:

The advantages to the practice would be that the nurse would be better equipped to undertake chronic disease monitoring (for example, run hypertension clinics), see minor illness in same day surgeries, give telephone advice and triage more efficiently, do home visits and prescribe her own dressings, medication and repeat prescriptions. This could result in the following:

1. A reduced work load for GPs.
2. A larger list size co-managed by GPs and nurse prescribers – increased income for the practice.
3. If there is difficulty in recruiting doctors, the shortfall may be safely filled by nurses capable of prescribing. The new GMS contract allows practices to employ nurses rather than additional partners when their list size increases – this has the potential for boosting practice profits.
4. Increased job satisfaction for GPs and nurses – morale is improved.
5. An improved standard of care for patients – studies (*BMJ* themed issue, (Volume 320, Issue 7241), 15 April 2000) show that nurses do not prescribe more than doctors and they offer a better quality of care to patients.
6. If nurses run the chronic disease and minor ailments clinics, then doctors can be freed to specialise in other aspects of care that were traditionally the domain of hospital consultants, hence the increase in GPs with Special Interests (GPwSIs).

- Do not support the nurse's application:

The disadvantages to the practice are:

1. The cost of training a nurse prescriber. This includes the cost of the course, locum cover for study days, and the extra burden of work facing the nurses who are left to cover her absence. Will all the nurses in the practice eventually want to be trained in prescribing?

2. Nurses are expensive to train and once trained may leave, taking their skills with them. They may stay if offered higher salaries.
3. Doctors may feel redundant and doctor morale in the surgery may decrease.
4. Doctors work faster. Nurses have longer consulting times and perform more investigations than doctors.
5. Are we allowing non-medically trained people to practice medicine? GPs have at least nine years of training and may be better equipped to diagnose unusual presentations and rare pathology. Nurse treatments tend to be protocol- and guideline-driven and difficult pathology and patient questioning may be beyond their ability.
6. Are we training nurses to do jobs that doctors no longer want to do, such as chronic disease management and care in inner cities?
7. The traditional doctor–patient relationship based on mutual knowledge and close rapport is under threat. There is less continuity of care, with the doctor only being accessed when difficulties arise.
8. Prescribing nurses will need to be supported and supervised. GPs may need to provide mentoring and advice, whereas new GP partners offer a wider skill set and are more autonomous.

Choice and justify. There is no right answer. One way in which the question can be answered is listed below.

I would support nurse prescribing because:

- The new GMS contract allows more flexible working patterns. The surgery can therefore replace a leaving partner, increase its list size, or do without a GP registrar / retainer by having a nurse who is able to prescribe independently. The initial training cost will be outweighed by the long-term benefits to the partnership. A contract with the nurse can be drawn up such that she gives a year of return of service and pays 50% of the training costs if she leaves earlier.
- The quality of patient care will be improved. Nurses will manage chronic diseases and minor ailments; doctors will offer new services locally. The GPs may be able to concentrate on more difficult patients and have time to develop enhanced services which are further remunerated under the new GMS contract.
- Quality and outcome targets may be easier to achieve.
- The morale of the PHCT will be improved.

Check and reflect:

Having made a decision to support the development of nurse prescribing within my practice, I would hope that audit of the nurse's work shows that:

- She is prescribing appropriately and within the nurse prescribers' formulary (see *BNF*, September 2004. www.bnf.org).
- She is seeing appropriate patients – chronic disease clinics, minor ailments, nursing home reviews.
- Her prescribing is in line with the partners – she is not prescribing more antibiotics for self-limiting ailments.

132

- Her prescribing is evidence-based and in line with local guidelines, for example trimethoprim as a first-line antibiotic for uncomplicated UTIs.
- The practice is achieving more Q and O points, particularly in chronic disease management.
- The doctor time saved by having a prescribing nurse has been put to good use – new doctor services have developed.
- A patient satisfaction survey shows that the patients are happy with the organisational changes.

LEARNING POINTS

- Nurse practitioners can undertake chronic disease monitoring, see minor illness in same day surgeries, triage
- Are nurse practitioners a cheaper non-medically trained resource?
- The nurse prescribers' formulary
- The difference between nurse prescribers and nurse practitioners (see below)

ADDITIONAL INFORMATION

From DoH website: http://www.dh.gov.uk/PolicyAndGuidance/ MedicinesPharmacyAndIndustry/Prescriptions/NursingPrescribing/fs/en

As of 2002, Extended Formulary nurses may prescribe a list of some 180 Prescription Only Medicines (plus all relevant Pharmacy and General Sales List medicines) to treat approximately 80 medical conditions.

The Nurse Prescribers' Extended Formulary includes six Controlled Drugs for pain relief.

Nurses are able to use Patient Group Directions for the supply and administration of Schedule 4 and Schedule 5 Controlled Drugs – with the exception of anabolic steroids. Nurses in accident and emergency departments and coronary units in hospitals may prescribe diamorphine for the treatment of cardiac pain.

In addition, the introduction of supplementary prescribing by nurses and pharmacists, following diagnosis by a doctor, will allow nurses trained in prescribing to prescribe for a range of chronic conditions and health needs, on the basis of an agreed patient-specific Clinical Management Plan.

No nurses will be required to undertake training for prescribing unless they wish to do so.

Nurse practitioners differ from nurse prescribers. See http://www.nursepractitioner.org.uk/. The first nurse practitioners qualified from the Royal College of Nursing Nurse Practitioner programme in 1992. The RCN defines the nurse practitioner as 'a registered nurse, who has undertaken a specific course of study of at least first degree (honours) level and who makes professionally autonomous decisions for which he or she is responsible. A nurse practitioner receives patients with undifferentiated and undiagnosed problems and makes an assessment of their health needs, based on highly developed nursing knowledge and skills, including skills not usually exercised by nurses, such as physical examination.'

Willis A and Maclaine K (2004) Just what is a nurse practitioner? *New Generalist*, **2**(2), 62–3.

Factors that have facilitated the development of the nurse practitioner include:

- the government's ambitious healthcare policy
- changing workforce demographics
- increased consumer demand

Cox C and Jones M (2000) An evaluation of the management of patients with sore throats by practice nurses and GPs. *British Journal of General Practice*, **50**, 872–876.

The aim of this UK-based observational study was to compare the quality of management of sore throats by practice nurses and GPs in a routine nursing triage system. A total of 44% of patients consulted the practice nurse and 56% consulted the GP. Severity of presenting illness was similar in the two groups.

- The reconsultation rates, antibiotic prescription, and dissatisfaction rates were the same for both groups.
- More patients seeing the practice nurse recalled receiving advice about home remedies (76% versus 54%).

Laurant MGH, Hermens RPMG *et al.* (2004) Impact of nurse practitioners on workload of general practitioners: randomised controlled trial. *BMJ*, **328**(7445), 927–30.

The objective of this Dutch study involving 48 GPs was to examine the impact on the GP's workload of adding nurse practitioners to the general practice team. Five nurses were randomly allocated to general practitioners to undertake specific elements of care according to agreed guidelines. The control group received no nurse. Outcomes were measured six months before and 18 months after the intervention.

Conclusion: Adding nurse practitioners to general practice teams did not reduce the workload of general practitioners, at least in the short term. This implies that nurse practitioners are used as supplements, rather than substitutes, for care given by general practitioners.

GP vacancies are taking longer to fill.

The Department of Health's *GP vacancy survey for England and Wales 2004* showed that it now takes 4.5 months to fill a GP vacancy, compared to 3.5 months in 2003.

Research from the University of York, published in *BJGP* in December 2004, shows that despite a 20% rise in GP recruitment in England over the last 18 years, there is still a shortage of GPs in underprivileged places, such as rural and deprived urban areas.

CONSULTATION MODELS

This brief overview of the common consultation models is based on *The consultation* by Pendleton *et al*. (2000).

WHAT IS A MEDICAL CONSULTATION?

The consultation is the medium through which medicine is frequently practised – it is the encounter between the patient and the doctor. Some encounters are satisfactory to both the patient and the doctor; others are unsatisfactory and dysfunctional to one or both parties. Researchers have studied these encounters from various perspectives:

- The medical perspective – this is concerned with diseases and diagnosis. The underlying assumption of the medical perspective is that illness and disease can be explained by changes to the structure or functioning of the body (pathophysiology). However, this rigorous scientific approach is limited – patients are not broken-down machines.
- The holistic perspective – this is concerned with placing the illness experience in physical, psychological and social contexts. The underlying assumption of the social perspective is that the understanding the patient has of what is happening to him as well as his emotional response to his illness define and determine the problem and its management. However, a danger with this model is that responsibility for the illness may be transferred to the doctor – the medicalisation of health.

In summary, 'disease' is the cause of sickness in terms of pathophysiology, whilst 'illness' is the patient's unique experience of sickness.

This chapter intends to present a brief overview of various consultation models. It will:

- Describe the model
- Discuss the assumptions made by the model
- Discuss evidence (if any) to support or refute these assumptions
- Discuss how the model has contributed to our understanding of the GP consultation.

THE BIOMEDICAL APPROACH

Description
Take an accurate and relevant history – observation
Perform an accurate and relevant examination – observation
Make a provisional diagnosis – hypothesis
Order and interpret the results of appropriate investigations – hypothesis testing
Make a definitive diagnosis – deduction

Assumptions made
- Every illness is caused by a definable agent (Robert Koch's postulate).
- Once the diagnosis is made in terms of this definable agent, a rational treatment is applied.

Evidence

Hampton *et al.* (1975) studied 80 patients and found that taking a good history made the diagnosis in 66 patients. Physical examination was useful in 7 patients; investigations were useful in 7 patients. The biomedical model places too much emphasis on examination and investigation.

Elstein *et al.* (1978) showed that clinicians do not follow the model in a step-wise manner – they generate hypotheses early on in the consultation and direct the consultation towards testing these hypotheses in turn.

Contributions

Positive
- In any single consultation the doctor may form, test and discard a large number of diagnostic hypotheses based on the information or cues he receives from the patient.
- The biomedical model proposes a rigorous scientific approach to problem-solving – such disciplined thinking has been responsible for good quality research and is the cornerstone of evidence-based medicine (EBM).

Limitations of the model
- It is reductionist – patients are seen and treated in terms of signs, symptoms and diagnoses and labelled accordingly.
- It is doctor-centred – there is no mention of the patient's feelings, beliefs, and opinions, any sharing of information or agreement of a management plan.
- The biomedical model is of limited value when an objective physical disorder cannot be diagnosed. The model may actually encourage further investigation of the patient until a 'disorder' is unearthed.
- The biomedical model de-emphasises the contribution of non-verbal communication.
- It omits the therapeutic use of the doctor–patient relationship.
- It fails to recognise that a consultation can be one of a series, as is often the case in general practice.

More modern consultation models have developed in response to these criticisms.

THE ANTHROPOLOGICAL APPROACH

Description

This model was developed from studying man's illness behaviour in different cultures.

A healing ritual consists of:

- giving the problem a name (diagnosis)
- performing a therapeutic ritual (management)
- renaming the problem as cured or improved (cure)

Patients believe healers. Society has invested the healers with authority (called Aesculapean authority) which derives from:

- the doctors' greater knowledge or expertise – sapiential authority
- the doctors' desire or motivation to do good – moral authority
- the doctors' desire to see the practice of medicine as something of a mystery – charismatic authority

Assumptions made
In the healing process, doctors and patients have roles. The patient assumes the more passive, recipient role and doctors assume the pro-active, responsive role which in turn is the source of their authority.

Evidence
The model is based on anthropological research done by Kleinman (1980), Osmond (1980) and Waitzkin and Stoekle (1976).

Contributions
Positive

- The anthropological model highlights the 'sick role' and 'healing role' adopted by patients and doctors.
- By virtue of their healing role, society invests doctors with authority.

Limitations of the model

- The anthropological model tells us about the social interaction between doctors and patients. However, the model may be criticised for dealing with the wider social context and is limited in its application to the individual context.

THE TRANSACTIONAL ANALYSIS APPROACH

Description
The human psyche consists of three ego states (Berne, 1964):

- the parent – commands, directs, prohibits, controls, nurtures
- the adult – sorts out information and works logically
- the child – intuition, creativity, spontaneity, enjoyment

At any point, each of us is in a state of mind where we think, feel, behave, react and have attitudes as if we were a parent (critical or caring), a logical adult or a child (spontaneous or dependent).

Assumptions
- Many general practice consultations are conducted between a parental doctor and a child-like patient. This interaction is not always in the best interests of either party.
- When transactions are repeated in a predictable way, for psychological benefit, they become games. One example is the 'yes but' game in which the patient produces reasons why a suggestion will not work, thereby relinquishing responsibility for the problem.

Evidence
The transactional model was based on the work of Berne (1964).

Contributions

Positive
- The transactional analysis model makes doctors aware of their patients' attempts to transfer responsibility to them.
- It also highlights the games people play and teaches doctors to break out of these cycles of behaviour.
- This model is particularly useful in analysing why communication breaks down during a consultation.

Limitations of the model
- Analysing the consultation in terms of Berne's model may be difficult and time-consuming.
- The transactional analysis model may make the doctor suspicious of his patients' motivation – consultations may be seen in terms of manipulative games.

BALINT'S APPROACH TO THE CONSULTATION

Description
- Psychological problems are often manifested physically and even physical disease has its own psychological consequences which need particular attention.
- Doctors have feelings and those feelings have a function in the consultation.
- Specific training is needed to change the doctor's behaviour so that he can become more sensitive to the patient.
- The 'drug doctor' is a term that describes the doctor's therapeutic contribution to the consultation. It describes the degree of efficacy of the doctor as a therapeutic intervention, as well as the doctor's unforeseen negative outcomes (side effects).
- The 'flash technique' – the doctor becomes aware of his feelings in the consultation, and when he interprets this back to the patient, the patient gains some insight into his problems.

Evidence

Michael Balint based his writing (*The doctor, his patient and the illness*, 1957) on his work with groups of doctors who regularly met to discuss their 'problem' cases.

Contributions

Positive
- The Balint model highlights the importance of treating bodies and minds simultaneously. It emphasises the contribution of psychological factors to the presenting illness.
- Doctors are seen as active participants in the consultation. In particular, doctors are encouraged to acknowledge their feelings and to feed these back to the patient so that the patient may develop insight into his problem. This is the first consultation model to stress the importance of the doctor's feelings.

Limitations of the model
- Doctors may indiscriminately feed back their feelings to all their patients – 'to Balint'.
- A great deal of emphasis is placed on intuition – this should complement, not replace, logic and reasoning.

BYRNE AND LONG (1976)

In 1976 Byrne and Long analysed approximately 2500 consultations from 71 GPs.

Description

Byrne and Long studied the verbal behaviour of doctors. They found that the doctor's consultation had 6 phases:

1. The doctor establishes a relationship with the patient.
2. The doctor attempts to discover or actually discovers the reasons for the patient's attendance.
3. The doctor conducts a verbal or physical examination or both.
4. The doctor and/or patient consider the condition.
5. The doctor and patient agree and detail further treatment or investigation if necessary.
6. The consultation is terminated (usually by the doctor).

The doctor's consultation style ranged from doctor-centred (based only on the doctor's knowledge) to patient-centred (incorporating the patient's experience). Dysfunctional consultations occurred when the doctor failed to discover the reason for the patient's attendance (2nd phase) or because the doctor did not tailor his explanation to his patient's beliefs (4th phase).

Assumptions
- The Byrne and Long (1976) model emphasises the contribution of verbal communication and downplays the contribution of non-verbal

communication. The criticism here is that a picture is worth a thousand words – doctors often judge the severity of a patient's chest pain not only by the words he uses to describe the pain, but also by his appearance – his breathlessness, sweating and writhing.

- The Byrne and Long (1976) model assumes that the content of the conversation is all-important. It underestimates the importance of the communication process – the tone of voice, facial expression and warmth of the doctor.

Evidence

Byrne and Long conducted field research. Their work on non-verbal communication was expanded on by (1976, 1977), Coope and Metcalfe (1979), Raynes (1980), Cartwright and Anderson (1981), Tuckett (1982) and Pendleton (1983).

Contributions

Positive
- Byrne and Long's model provides a practical approach to addressing individual dysfunctional consultations.
- They recommend that doctors be taught how to discover their patients' beliefs about their problems and to tailor their explanations of illness to incorporate these beliefs.

Limitations of the model
- Verbal communication is disproportionately emphasised. Attention must also be paid to the process of communication, including non-verbal communication.

PENDLETON *ET AL.* (2003)

In *The consultation* (2003), Pendleton *et al.* propose a task-based approach to effective consulting. These tasks are derived from the needs of the patient, the aims of the doctor, the desired outcomes and the evidence that links them.

Description
The seven tasks of the GP consultation

1. To understand the reasons for the patient's attendance, including:
   - The patient's problem: its nature, history, aetiology and effects
   - The patient's perspective: their personal and social circumstances; ideas and values about health; their ideas about the problem, its causes and its management; their concerns about the problem and its implications; their expectations for information, involvement and care.
2. Taking into account the patient's perspective, to achieve a shared understanding:
   - About the problem
   - About the evidence and options for management

3. To enable the patient to choose an appropriate action for each problem:
   - Consider options and implications
   - Choose the most appropriate course of action
4. To enable the patient to manage the problem:
   - Discuss the patient's ability to take appropriate actions
   - Agree doctor and patient actions and responsibilities
   - Agree targets, monitoring and follow-up
5. To consider other problems:
   - Not yet presented
   - Continuing problems
   - At-risk factors
6. To use time appropriately:
   - In the consultation
   - In the longer term

To establish or maintain a relationship with the patient that helps to achieve the other tasks.

Assumptions
- The Pendleton model assumes that consulting is effective if it is patient-centred. There are two main problems with this assumption. First, how do we measure effectiveness – patient satisfaction, disease-based outcome criteria, doctor satisfaction, or fewer follow-up appointments? Secondly, does 'patient-centredness' actually improve the doctor's effectiveness?

Mead and Bower (2000) defined patient-centredness as:

1. understanding the biopsychosocial context in which the problem presents
2. appreciating the individual patient's experience of the illness
3. sharing the power within the relationship to maintain joint responsibility
4. recognising the effect of the relationship on the illness and maximising the benefits of the therapeutic alliance
5. recognising the doctor as a person and appreciating the impact of the doctor as an individual on the relationship.

Evidence
The task model is based on an analysis of the relevant literature, field research and the practical experience of the authors.

Contributions

Positive
- The recommendation for each of the seven tasks is evidence-based.
- The model is easy to teach and easy to use. A doctor can analyse the effectiveness of his consulting by reviewing his consultations against the suggested criteria. He is then able to identify the reasons for the dysfunctional consultation and take steps to improve his consulting technique – the model is practical.

- By focusing on the tasks, the feelings of the patient and the doctor can be relatively neglected.
- By reducing the complex behaviour of consulting into the completion of 7 tasks, the doctor's consultation is in danger of being converted into a tick-box exercise.
- The doctor is expected to complete each task proficiently, sensitively and smoothly within the allocated time – a rather daunting task in itself!
- Doctors have a set of beliefs that underpin their core values. If their fundamental beliefs about patients and medicine do not change, it is quite likely that task-based changes to their consulting behaviour will remain superficial and short-lived.

NEIGHBOUR (1987)

In *The inner consultation* (1987), Neighbour proposed that there are five important checkpoints along the consultation journey.

Description

The five checkpoints are:

- Connecting
- Summarising
- Handing over
- Safety netting
- Housekeeping

Connecting refers to establishing and maintaining a non-threatening relationship with the patient to achieve a level of rapport.

Summarising refers to taking a comprehensive history and reflecting this back to the patient. This ensures that both doctor and patient have reached a common, shared understanding of the presenting complaint – the physical problem as well as the patient's ideas, concerns and expectations of the illness and its management.

Handing over refers to the transfer of responsibility for management back to the patient. The doctor and the patient may well have different objectives for the consultation; the negotiation and handing over the consultation may involve some degree of compromise on both sides.

Safety netting refers to providing the patient with information on what to expect and what to do if they do not improve. General practice has been described as the art of managing the uncertain and provision needs to be made within the consultation for this. Patients will feel more secure if they have a clear outline of what to expect from their treatment and under what circumstances to re-consult.

Housekeeping refers to the doctor attending his own feelings, particularly those brought about by a consultation. If the emotions engendered by the consultation are not acknowledged and dealt with, they may spill over into the next. Sometimes, acknowledging these concerns may be all that is required.

Occasionally, the doctor needs to reflect on a consultation and possibly consider how to handle things differently in the future. In this way, the doctor learns from his practice.

Assumptions

The Neighbour model assumes that through good communication, it is possible for the doctor and patient to reach a shared understanding of the presenting problem. The counter argument is that you can bring a horse to water but you can't make it drink. Reaching a shared understanding is a two way process – the patient must have some understanding, insight and a willingness to modify his health beliefs. It is the doctor's responsibility to enter into the negotiation and to do so in language the patient understands. However, the overall responsibility for reaching a 'shared understanding' cannot be the doctor's alone. To assume sole responsibility invites 'medicalisation' of social problems.

Evidence

The Neighbour model is a theory on consultation and communication based on the practical experience of the author and informed by his reading of the medical, educational and philosophical literature.

Contributions

Positive

Other consultation models have already discussed ways of integrating the medical and holistic perspectives. Neighbour introduced the concepts of safety netting and housekeeping. Housekeeping is built on Balint's concept of the doctor's emotions having a useful purpose in the consultation. Where Balint advised doctors to reflect these feelings back to their patients to develop the patients' insight into the problem, Neighbour advises doctors to reflect on their feelings to develop their own insight into their strengths and weaknesses as doctors. By developing self-awareness, doctors can improve as clinicians – they can, in the words of Neighbour, 'develop an effective and intuitive learning style'.

Limitations of the model
- When safety netting, doctors are in danger of slipping into a prescriptive consultation style if they assume a parent–child approach.
- Sometimes, because of the doctor's fears and insecurities over medico-legal concerns, safety netting transforms from a tool to manage uncertainty into a technique for practising defensive medicine.

ADDITIONAL INFORMATION

Freeman GK, Horder JP, Howie JGR, Hungin AP, Hill AP, Shah NC, and Wilson A (2002) Evolving general practice consultation in Britain: issues of length and context. *BMJ*, **324,** 880–882.

Kravitz RL and Melnikow J (2001) Engaging patients in medical decision making. *BMJ*, **323,** 584–585.

Little P, Everitt H, Williamson I, Warner G, Moore M, Gould C, Ferrier K, and Payne S (2001) Observational study of effect of patient centredness and positive approach on outcomes of general practice consultations. *BMJ*, **323,** 908–911.

Little P, Everitt H, Williamson I, Warner G, Moore M, Gould C, Ferrier K, and Payne S (2001) Preferences of patients for patient centred approach to consultation in primary care: observational study. *BMJ*, **322,** 468.

McKinstry B (2000) Do patients wish to be involved in decision making in the consultation? A cross sectional survey with video vignettes. *BMJ*, **321,** 867–871.

Stewart M (2001) Towards a global definition of patient centred care. *BMJ*, **322,** 444–445.

Walter J and Bayat A (2003) Neurolinguistic programming: verbal communication. *BMJ*, **326,** 83.

RELEVANT LITERATURE

Bain JD (1976) **Doctor–patient communication in general practice consultations.** *Medical Education*, **10,** 125–31.

Bain JD (1977) **Patient knowledge and the content of the consultation in general practice.** *Medical Education*, **11,** 347–50.

Balint M (1957) **The doctor, his patient and the illness.** *Pitman*, London.

Berne E (1964) **Games people play.** *Penguin*, Harmondsworth.

Byrne PS and Long BEL (1976) **Doctors talking to patients.** *HMSO*, London.

Cartwright A and Anderson R (1981) **General practice revisited.** *Tavistock*, London.

Coope J and Metcalfe D (1979) **How much do patients know?** *Journal of Royal College of General Practitioners,* **29**, 482–8.

Elstein AS, Shulman LS, and Sprafha SA (1978) **Medical problem solving: an analysis of clinical reasoning.** *Harvard University Press,* Cambridge, MA.

Hampton JR, Harrison MJE, Mitchell JRA, Pritchard JS, and Seymour C (1975) **Relative contributions of history taking, physical examination and laboratory investigation to diagnosis and management of medical outpatients.** *BMJ,* **ii**, 486–9.

Kleinman A (1980) **Patients and healers in the context of culture.** *University of California Press,* Berkeley.

Mead N and Bower P (2000) **Patient centredness: a conceptual framework and review of the empirical literature.** *Soc. Sci. Med.,* **51**, 1087–110.

Neighbour R (1987) **The inner consultation: how to develop an effective and intuitive consulting style.** *MTP Press,* Lancaster.

Osmond H (1980) **God and the doctor.** *New England Journal of Medicine,* **302**, 555–8.

Pendleton DA (1983) **Doctor–patient communication: a review. In Doctot–patient communication** (editors Pendleton DA and Haslar JC). *Academic Press.*

Pendleton D, Schofield T, Tate P and Havelock P (2000) **The consultation: an approach to learning and teaching.** *Oxford University Press,* Oxford.

Pendleton D, Schofield T, Tate P and Havelock P (2003) **The new consultation: developing doctor–patient communication.** *Oxford University Press,* Oxford.

Raynes NV (1980) **A preliminary study of search procedures and patient management techniques in general practice.** *Journal of Royal College of General Practitioners,* **13**, 166–72.

Silverman J, Kurtz S and Draper J (1998) **Skills for communicating with patients.** *Radcliffe Medical Press,* Oxon.

Stott NCH and Davis RH (1979) **The exceptional potential in each primary care consultation.** *Journal of the Royal College of General Practitioners,* **29,** 201–5.

Tate P (2003) **The doctor's communication handbook.** 4th Edition. *Radcliffe Medical Press,* Oxon.

Tuckett D (ed) (1976) **An introduction to medical sociology.** *Tavistock,* London.

Waitzkin and Stoekle (1976) **The communication of information about illness: clinical, social and methodological considerations.** *Advanced Journal of Psychosomatic Medicine,* **8**, 180–215.

CLINICAL GOVERNANCE

Clinical governance (CG) is unlikely to be asked as a direct question. However, an understanding of CG is needed to answer questions regarding the quality of care in the NHS. Questions such as 'What do you understand by quality assurance and accountability in the NHS?' and 'How could GPs improve their delivery of care to patients?' all link up with the concept of CG.

CG is a complex concept. This chapter tries to explain the concept simply; a comprehensive discussion would take an entire book! Complicated questions can be answered using a simple format called the '**5 Ws and 1 H**': what, when, why, where, who and how.

WHAT IS CG?

'A framework through which NHS organisations are accountable for continuously improving the *quality* of their services and safeguarding high standards of care by creating an environment in which excellence in clinical care will flourish'
A first class service (DoH, 1998)

The DoH defined *quality* as doing the right things, to the right people, at the right time.

CG aims to evaluate the quality of medical practice against agreed standards and to remedy any gaps identified in routine practice.

'Putting quality at the top of the NHS agenda will ensure fair access to effective, prompt, high quality care wherever a patient is treated in the NHS'
A first class service (DoH, 1998)

WHEN WAS CG INTRODUCED?

The NHS introduced the concept of clinical governance in 1998.

WHERE WILL CG BE INTRODUCED?

Improvements are needed at every level of the NHS, from GP surgeries to national structures (hence the introduction of NSFs, NICE, and the Modernisation Agency).

WHAT NEEDS IMPROVING?

Improvements can be made to:

- the physical components of the NHS – the surgery buildings, practice equipment, patient records and the practice team.
- the care given to patients and carers – are we following best practice?
- the outcomes of the treatment given – are we improving morbidity and mortality?

A criteria-based approach is a good objective way of measuring and achieving quality. The RCGP Quality Practice Award (QPA) and the new GMS contract provide a ready-made set of criteria that can be used locally.

WHY IS IMPROVEMENT NEEDED?

- The public has lost faith in the health service following the Bristol, Alder Hay and Shipman scandals.
- There is increased consumerism – people demand high quality care.
- The government spends a large proportion of the budget on health – it wants an accountable NHS.

The public and government both want a high quality, accountable and transparent health service. Within the context of general practice, CG is about *assuring quality*:

- reducing the variation in the delivery of care by different GPs,
- setting agreed targets for improvement,
- systematically meeting targets.

CG in primary care is also about *assuring accountability* – demonstrating to patients, members of the PHCT, the PCT and the government that standards are satisfactory and are being achieved.

HOW WILL WE MAKE THESE IMPROVEMENTS?

Improvements within the practice will take place by:

- practising evidence-based medicine – assessing clinical information on the internet from desktops; making clinical guidelines available electronically.
- disseminating good practice – copying letters to patients, sharing clinical 'titbits' with colleagues electronically and at meetings.
- adopting quality improvement processes – undertaking audits regularly, updating the practice drug formulary, participating in primary care collaborative projects.
- using data appropriately – auditing chronic disease management, analysing prescribing data, working with local pharmacists to review patients on regular medication.
- reducing clinical risk – by having regular significant event meetings.
- learning lessons from complaints – holding multidisciplinary meetings to reflect on and learn from complaints.

- tackling poor performance – undertaking annual resuscitation training, lengthening the appointment times for doctors who regularly over-run.
- continuing professional development – using staff PDPs, staff appraisal and 360 degree feedback.
- developing leadership – defining the roles of the CG partner and nursing representative.

These initiatives are known as the Ten Commandments of CG (Van Zwanenberg and Harrison, 2003).

DOES CG WORK? WHAT DO WE EVALUATE?

There is currently little published evidence that clinical governance makes any measurable difference.

When Degeling *et al.* (2004) reviewed CG in practice, they thought that CG should be a bottom-up (not top-down) activity – there should be less emphasis on inspection and performance management. The top-down model is flawed and should be replaced by a model that asks the following questions:

- **Are we doing the right things?** Given assessed health needs and existing resource constraints, are we delivering value for money? For common conditions, how appropriate and effective are the services we offer?
- **Are we doing things right?** Are we managing clinical performance according to national codes of clinical practice? For common conditions, how systematised are our care processes and how are we performing on risk, safety, quality, patient evaluation and clinical outcomes?
- **Are we keeping up with new developments** and what are we doing to extend our capacity to undertake clinical work in these areas? What strategies are in place for service and professional development for each condition? What are we doing about clinical mentoring, leadership development and staff appraisals?

HOW WILL WE DELIVER AND SUPPORT THE CULTURAL CHANGES NEEDED?

A number of NHS and DoH organisations are working to improve quality in the NHS. Dr Tim Wilson, writing for the National Electronic Library for Health, identifies the following agencies:

- *National Patient Safety Agency* – making the NHS safer for patients
- *National Institute for Clinical Excellence* – telling us what to do (and sometimes what not to do)
- *Commission for Health Improvement* – the independent watchdog that reports to Parliament on the performance of Trusts in England and Wales
- *National Clinical Assessment Authority* – helps local organisations with the assessment of doctors whose performance gives concern

- *Modernisation Agency* – the body charged with modernising care across the NHS. Within the Mod Agency (as it is known) are a number of teams including
  - ○ *Clinical Governance Support Team* – doing just that
  - ○ *National Primary Care Development Team* – working on a number of large improvement projects nationally and regionally to improve amongst other things, access and coronary heart disease care
  - ○ *Leadership Centre* – helping to create more leaders in the NHS
  - ○ *National PCT Development team* (known as NatPaCT) – helping to build the capabilities of Primary Care Trusts
  - ○ *Changing workforce programme*
  - ○ *Service Improvement* (formerly NPAT)

WHO ARE THE KEY PLAYERS?

The Labour Government discussed CG in '*A first class service: quality in the new NHS*'. Liam Donaldson wrote a key paper about the introduction of CG to the NHS (*BMJ*, 1998) and Neville Goodman (speaking for many doctors) wrote a critique of this paper.

CG appears in Annex B of the new contract (number 21) as a statutory and contractual requirement. This states that:

- All practices should have a system of CG to enable quality assurance, quality improvement and enhanced patient safety.
- There should be a nominated clinical governance lead in each practice.
- CG should be embedded in all the structures underpinning practice.

LEARNING POINTS

- Assuring quality and accountability
- The Ten Commandments of CG
- Evaluation: doing the right things, doing things right, keeping up to date?
- *A first class service: quality in the new NHS*
- Annex B of the new contract (number 21)

ADDITIONAL INFORMATION

Goodman NW (1998). Clinical Governance. Sacred cows: to the abattoir. *BMJ*, **317**, 1725–1727. Neville Goodman writes:

'I have read "Clinical governance and the drive for quality improvement in the new NHS in England" carefully, word by word, and some parts several times. I have tried to understand why they needed over four pages to impart the commonsense message that we must all strive after quality in practising medicine;

I have retained little beyond that it is our statutory duty now to provide quality in our medical care. The essay is all thought and no action, an epitome of hope over expectation, a high sounding clarion call of wonderful things just over the horizon. Most depressing of all, the authors seem to recognise the real difficulties but ignore just how obdurate these difficulties are. The result is an essay full of the "what" but short on the "how."'

Marshall M *et al.* (2002) A qualitative study of cultural changes in PCOs needed to implement clinical governance. *British Journal of General Practice*, **52**(481), 641–645.

The aim of this qualitative study was to investigate the importance of culture and cultural change for the implementation of clinical governance in general practice by PCGs / PCTs, to identify perceived desirable and undesirable cultural facilitators and barriers to changing culture. Results: The most desirable cultural traits were the value placed on a commitment to public accountability by the practices, their willingness to work together and learn from each other, and the ability to be self-critical and learn from mistakes. The main barriers to cultural change were the high level of autonomy of practices and the perceived pressure to deliver rapid measurable changes in general practice.

Campbell S (2001) Improving the quality of care through clinical governance. *BMJ*, **322**(7302), 1580–1582.

Primary care groups and trusts are responsible for implementing clinical governance, including monitoring and improving the quality of care. In their first two years they have concentrated on educating and supporting health professionals and encouraging shared learning. Information about the quality of care provided in general practice is shared between practices and with the public, offered in a form that permits practices to be identified. Many groups and trusts are offering incentives to practices to promote improvement in the quality of care. Sanctions and disciplinary action are rarely used when dealing with poor performance. Limited resources and the pace of change are potential obstacles to future success in improving the quality of care.

Pringle M (2000) Participating in clinical governance. *BMJ*, **321**(7263), 737–740.

Clinical governance is intended to improve standards of care and at the same time to protect the public from unacceptable care. The move from continuing medical education for doctors to continuing professional development for the whole primary care team presents new challenges for multidisciplinary learning and performance monitoring. To deal with poor performance, clinical governance leaders will need skills to assess the nature of the problem, educational resources to deal with it, and managerial resources to facilitate the process.

Allen P (2000) Accountability for clinical governance: developing collective responsibility for quality in primary care. *BMJ*, **321**(7261), 608–611.

Clinical governance in primary care is aimed at enhancing the collective responsibility and accountability of professionals in primary care trusts. It is mainly concerned with increasing accountability of primary care professionals to local communities (downwards accountability), the NHS hierarchy (upwards accountability), and their peers (horizontal accountability). Limited resources are likely to ensure that upwards accountability is given priority.

Rosen R (2000) Improving quality in the changing world of primary care. *BMJ*, **321**(7260), 551–554.

Clinical governance in primary care must focus on individual patients and whole populations; this creates tensions between a view of good practice based on individual rights and a population approach focused on the distribution of services.

RELEVANT LITERATURE

Journal articles
Degeling P *et al.* (1998) **Do professional subcultures set limits to hospital reform.** *Clinician in management*, **7**, 89–98.
Pringle M, Bradley C, Carmichael CM *et al.* (1995) **Significant event auditing: a study of the feasibility and potential of case based auditing in primary medical care.** Occasional paper no. 70. *RCGP Publications*.
Scally G, Donaldson LJ (1998) **Looking forward: clinical governance and the drive for quality improvement in the new NHS in England.** BMJ, **317**, 61–5.

Books
Van Zwanenberg T and Harrison J (editors) (2003) **Clinical Governance in Primary Care.** 2nd edition. *Radcliffe Medical Press*, Oxford.

Internet
- http://www.nelh.nhs.uk/quality/
- http://www.doh.gov.uk/clinicalgovernance
- http://www.rsm.ac.uk/pub/cgb.htm
- Roland M and Baker R (1999) **Clinical governance: a practical guide for primary care teams**. *National Primary Care Research and Development,* Manchester.
  http://www.npcrdc.man.ac.uk/publications/handbook%20clinical%20governance.pdf
- Secretary of State for Health. (1998) **A first class service. Quality in the new NHS**. NHS Executive, Leeds. www.nhshistory.net/a_first_class_service.htm

PATIENT SAFETY

WHY DO I NEED TO KNOW ABOUT PATIENT SAFETY FOR THE MRCGP EXAM?

It is a current hot topic. The oral exam tests the doctor's professional values and care of patients. Patient safety is an important component of the Clinical Governance (CG) agenda. CG has changed the way in which we deliver care to patients. The aim is to give safe, high quality care. A question on patient safety may appear in many guises, such as:

- What mechanisms should GP practices have in place to reduce mistakes?
- A practice nurse has given an incorrect vaccine. How would you manage this situation?
- You notice that the diclofenac injection you are about to give to a terminally ill patient is out of date. What steps will you take to prevent this from happening again in the future?

WHY IS PATIENT SAFETY IMPORTANT IN GENERAL PRACTICE?

- Non-maleficence is a key component of our professional ethics.
- Society expects good quality, safe care.
- Patient safety is an integral part of the CG agenda.
- Doctors are remunerated for having systems in place to reduce the risk of harm to their patients and to learn lessons from mistakes that were made. For example, four Q and O points are given if the practice undertakes six significant event reviews in the past three years.

HOW ARE PATIENTS HARMED BY HEALTHCARE PROFESSIONALS?

1. **Unavoidable risks** in medicine (some adverse events are inevitable)
   - Risks of medication (risk of a seizure with anti-malarials) or
   - Risks of treatment (risk of uterine perforation with the insertion of an IUD).

   Patients need to be warned about the possible harms and benefits of treatments in order to make informed choices. Good record-keeping is also important.

2. **Avoidable risks**

   These usually occur as a result of genuine mistakes. Research has suggested that around 10 per cent of patients admitted to UK acute hospitals suffer some kind of patient safety incident. Up to half of these mistakes may have been preventable. Systems should be designed to minimise such mistakes.

For example, analysis of reported incidents involving intrathecal chemotherapy injections resulted in changes to the design of the delivery system.

3. Criminal doctors

This constitutes a very small proportion of patient harm. Unfortunately Shipman will be remembered for a long time by the public.

4. Underperforming doctors

Doctors have a professional duty to maintain good medical practice and to keep up to date. Doctors may be underperforming because:

- They become deskilled (some GPs who became deskilled at providing intra-partum care withdrew these services)
- Doctors fail to provide up-to-date treatments which evidence-based research has shown to be effective. For example, failure to treat hypertension aggressively results in increased morbidity.
- Some doctors have poor diagnostic skills and behaviour (poor prescribing and referral patterns).

ADDRESSING AVOIDABLE RISK

The NHS intends to learn from the airline industry. The National Patient Safety Agency (NPSA) was formed following the publication of two reports on patient safety:

- *An organisation with a memory* (DoH, 2000), and its follow-up
- *Building a safer NHS for patients* (DoH, 2001).

The NPSA was tasked with developing:

- A **blame-free culture** – this will encourage doctors to openly discuss mistakes – theirs, their colleagues' and those due to the system in which they work. Staff who find themselves in a dysfunctional or repressive organisation will continue to be protected by whistleblowing legislation.
- A **national mechanism** for reporting and analysing risk. This aims to tackle the root cause of the risk. The NPSA is developing the National Reporting and Learning System (NRLS).
- Summary:

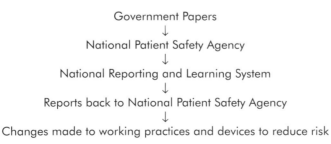

Government Papers
↓
National Patient Safety Agency
↓
National Reporting and Learning System
↓
Reports back to National Patient Safety Agency
↓
Changes made to working practices and devices to reduce risk

MECHANISMS FOR REPORTING RISK

NHS staff, patients and their carers will be able to report any patient safety incidents or near misses to the NRLS electronically. The NRLS has been designed to complement local systems, such as significant event reporting. The information they provide will be fed to the National Patient Safety Agency. The NPSA will:

- *collect and analyse* information on adverse events;
- *assimilate* other safety-related information from a variety of existing reporting systems and other sources in the UK and abroad;
- *learn lessons* and ensure that they are fed back into practice,
- where risks are identified, produce *solutions to prevent harm and specify national goals.*

RESPONDING TO THE HARM

At present, when there has been a failure of the service, a range of responses occurs. In future there will be two ways of responding – an independent investigation commissioned by either the Department of Health or by the Commission for Health Improvement.

WHAT CAN BE DONE LOCALLY TO REDUCE PATIENT HARM?

The National Patient Safety Agency has issued a guide to NHS staff – *Seven steps to patient safety* (2003). It sets out the seven steps that NHS organisations should take to improve patient safety.

- Build a safety culture – create a culture that is open and fair.
- Lead and support your staff – establish a clear and strong focus on patient safety throughout your organisation.
- Integrate your risk management activity – develop systems and processes to manage your risks and identify and assess things that could go wrong.
- Promote reporting – ensure your staff can easily report incidents locally and nationally.
- Involve and communicate with patients and the public – develop ways to communicate openly with patients.
- Learn and share safety lessons – encourage staff to use root cause analysis to learn how and why adverse incidents occurred.
- Implement solutions to prevent harm.

RISK MANAGEMENT IN GENERAL PRACTICE

Clinical risk management aims to identify, assess and then reduce risk to patients. The most common errors in general practice are due to administrative failures, such as errors in taking and passing on messages (31%). Treatment failures account for 23% of errors.

HOW DO GENERAL PRACTICES REDUCE THEIR RISK?

Practice equipment – a named individual should be responsible for regularly monitoring, maintaining and calibrating equipment. Drugs and vaccinations should be stored at the correct temperature.

Staff training – good induction and regular training should occur in manual handling, confidentiality issues, filing results and dealing with violent patients.

Health and safety – the practice should have a policy in place to deal with fire drills, the disposal of sharps, sterilising equipment and vaccination against hepatitis B.

Record-keeping – good notes are essential: they may form the GP's defence against a complaint.

Clinical guidelines – evidence-based guidelines should be easily available (preferably on desktops) and should be regularly updated.

Confidentiality and consent – practice staff must be made aware of the strict rules governing confidentiality. Patients should not be able to view the notes or overhear discussions about other patients. Practices should have appropriate consent forms for minor surgery, immunisations and other procedures.

Complaints – the practice should have an agreed procedure for handling patients' complaints. This should comply with the NHS procedures, and should be outlined in the practice leaflet.

Audit and significant event analysis – lessons learnt should improve patient care.

Adverse incident reporting – practices should have a mechanism for identifying and reporting adverse or significant events to the NPSA.

LEARNING POINTS

- Patients are harmed by avoidable errors, unavoidable errors, criminal doctors and underperforming doctors
- National Patient Safety Agency was formed to develop a blame-free culture and a national mechanism for reporting risk
- *Seven steps to patient safety* (2003)
- Audit and significant event analysis – learning lessons and improving care

---

ADDITIONAL INFORMATION

Quality indicators in the new GMS contract – a few examples are listed below.

4 points	There is a record of all practice-employed clinical staff having attended training / updating in basic life-support skills in the preceding 18 months
3 points	All new staff receive induction training
4 points	The practice has undertaken a minimum of 12 SEAs in the past three years which include (if these have occurred): • Any deaths occurring in the practice premises • Two new cancer diagnoses • Two deaths where terminal care has taken place at home • One patient complaint • One suicide • One section under the Mental Health Act
3 points	The practice has systems in place to ensure regular and appropriate inspection, calibration, maintenance and replacement of equipment including: • A defined responsible person • Clear recording • Systematic pre-planned schedules • Reporting of faults

RELEVANT LITERATURE

The complaints procedure is available at:
> www.doh.gov.uk/complaints/pbp-gps.pdfandn
> www.nhs.uk/patientsvoice/how_to_complain.asp

Confidentiality regulations and guidance are at: www.nhsia.nhs.uk/confidentiality

Consent forms are at: www.doh.gov.uk/consent/guidance.htm

Data protection help is available at: www.dataprotection.gov.uk with specific advice on the use and disclosure of health data at:
> www.dataprotection.gov.uk/dpr/dpdoc.nsf

Information about storing vaccines and temperature controls is at: www.pharmj.com/noticeboard/info/pip/lowtemperature.htmln www.rcn.org.uk

The Health and Safety Executive website is found at: www.hse.gov.uk, with further information about infection control available at:
> www.nhsplus.nhs.uk/nhsstaff/infection.asp

EVIDENCE-BASED MEDICINE

WHY DO I NEED TO KNOW ABOUT EVIDENCE-BASED MEDICINE FOR THE MRCGP EXAM?

The oral exam tests the doctor's personal and professional growth and his ability to provide up-to-date, effective care to his patients. A question on EBM may appear as:

- Name three medical websites that you use regularly.
- How do you know that you are managing heart failure well in general practice?
- Do you think that EBM has improved the quality of care in general practice?

WHY IS EBM IMPORTANT IN GENERAL PRACTICE?

Practice could be improved if practitioners were more familiar with the results of research. Doctors need to be able to access the literature, appraise papers for their validity and value and then convert their learning into practice that benefits their patients.

WHAT IS EBM?

EMB is a systematic approach to clinical decision-making. It involves:

- framing a focused question
- searching thoroughly for research-derived evidence
- appraising the evidence for its validity and relevance
- seeking and incorporating the user's values and preferences
- evaluating effectiveness through planned review against agreed success criteria.

It is based on similar principles to audit and performance review.

1. Framing a focused question:
Use the SMART principle to focus the question. The question must cover four areas:

- the patient or problem,
- the intervention being considered,
- the alternative intervention where appropriate and
- the outcome.

For example, in the question 'Do broad-spectrum antibiotics reduce the duration of pain and fever in acute, purulent OM in children aged 2 to 12 years?' the patient is a child between the ages of 2 and 12; the intervention is a broad-spectrum antibiotic; the alternative is treatment without antibiotics; the outcomes are duration of pain and fever.

2. Searching for the evidence

Searches can be done manually by trawling through textbooks and journals but these sources rapidly become outdated. Electronic databases are a reliable alternative. A good starting point is Medline and the Cochrane library. Other useful online databases include Bandolier, Best Evidence and General Practice Notebook (www.gpnotebook.co.uk). Searches can be done by the practitioner or by a medical librarian.

3. Appraising the evidence

Doctors apply their critical reading principles to understand the research. On first glance, doctors need to ascertain:

- whether the trial is valid,
- what the results are,
- whether the results are applicable locally.

To make these decisions, doctors need to understand, amongst other things, the concepts of P-values, confidence intervals, bias, confounding factors, intention to treat analysis, numbers needed to treat (NNT) and numbers needed to harm (NTH).

4. Incorporating the user's values

Using the example of otitis media, the research will not be applied to every child irrespective of their circumstances. Professional judgement is exercised in the application of research findings to clinical practice.

> 'Focusing too much on the rational and quantitative aspects of clinical problems – an inherent danger in EBM – can have a negative influence on the doctor–patient relationship and can erode the caregivers' role in providing care in fullest and most human way possible . . . Evidence is not enough: we need to communicate with our patients, listen to their concerns, elicit their values, be involved, really care about them. We also need to integrate the evidence with patients' values and preferences.'
>
> (Hunink, 2004)

5. Evaluating the effectiveness against agreed success criteria

EBM is about incorporating research evidence into clinical practice. How will doctors know if the changes they introduced improved the health of their patients? The final step involves assessing the usefulness of the intervention. For example, did the reduction in antibiotic prescribing in OM lead to more follow-up consultations, greater use of the out of hours service, or result in a higher complication rate? Did many patients complain about the new practice?

Evidence is classified according to the strength of the study design.

Grade 1	Strong evidence from at least one published meta-analysis / systematic review of multiple well-designed randomised controlled trials (RCT)
Grade 2	Strong evidence from at least one RCT of appropriate size and in an appropriate clinical setting
Grade 3	Evidence from published well-designed trials without randomisation, single group pre-post, cohort, time series or matched case-controlled studies
Grade 4	Evidence from well-designed non-experimental studies from more than one centre or research group
Grade 5	Opinions of respected authorities, based on clinical evidence, descriptive studies or reports of expert consensus committees

The hierarchy of EBM may be misleading. Hunink (2004) writes that a systematic review of a few small, poorly-conducted trials is clearly not better than one large, well-done, double-blind trial. Randomisation is not always ethically justifiable. Some information such as the treatment of fractures with plaster casts comes from observational data (grade 5 evidence).

WHAT DO GPs THINK ABOUT EBM?

Most GPs believe that EBM will improve their practice but many do not know how to conduct a search. In a 1998 survey of 450 Wessex GPs, fewer than half were aware of the Cochrane Database of Systematic Reviews and less than a quarter had access to Medline at their surgeries (McColl *et al.*, 1998).

HOW OFTEN DO GPs NEED TO LOOK FOR FURTHER INFORMATION?

It has been estimated that GPs experience areas of uncertainty that raise questions about their practice at least once every 15 patients (Ely *et al.*, 1992).

LEARNING POINTS

- The five steps of EBM
- Electronic databases: Cochrane, Medline
- Use professional judgement to incorporate the users' values
- The hierarchy of EBM (Grades 1 to 5)
- GPs experience uncertainty once every 15 patients

ADDITIONAL INFORMATION

The READER method of critical reading (McAuley, 1994) sets out some basic rules to help GPs discriminate between useful and less useful reading.

- First, GPs should read those articles that are relevant to their daily work.
- Secondly, the article should tell GPs something new.
- Thirdly, GPs should be able to apply the knowledge in their practice.

Criteria	Possible score	Actual score (tick)
Relevance: 1. not relevant to general practice 2. allied to general practice 3. only relevant to specialised general practice 4. broadly relevant to all general practice 5. relevant to me subtotal	1 2 3 4 5 ☐	
Education: 1. would certainly not influence behaviour 2. could possibly influence behaviour 3. would cause reconsideration of behaviour 4. would probably alter behaviour 5. would definitely change behaviour subtotal	1 2 3 4 5 ☐	
Applicability 1. impossible in my practice 2. fundamental changes needed 3. perhaps possible 4. could be done with reorganisation 5. I could do that tomorrow subtotal	1 2 3 4 5 ☐	
Discrimination 1. poor descriptive study 2. moderately good descriptive study 3. good descriptive study by methods not reproducible 4. good descriptive study with sound methodology 5. single-blind study with attempts to control 6. controlled single-blind study 7. double-blind controlled study with method problem 8. double-blind controlled study with statistical deficiency 9. sound scientific paper with minor faults 10. scientifically sound paper subtotal	1 2 3 4 5 6 7 8 9 10 ☐	
total		

The READER model (McAuley, 1994).

RELEVANT LITERATURE

BMJ (30 October 2004, volume 329) is a themed issue dealing with EBM.

Ely JW, Burch RJ, Vinson DC (1992) **The information needs of family physicians: case-specific clinical questions.** *Journal of Family Practice*, **35,** 265–9.

Fowkes FGR, Fulton PM (1991) **Critical appraisal of published research: introductory guidelines.** *BMJ*, **302,** 1136–40.

Hunink MGM (2004) **Does evidence based medicine do more good than harm?** *BMJ*, **329,** 1051.

McAuley D (1994) **READER: an acronym to aid critical reading in general practice.** *British Journal of General Practice*, **44,** 83–85.

McColl A, Smith H, White P, Field J (1998) **General practitioners' perceptions of the route to evidence based medicine: a questionnaire survey.** *BMJ*, **316** (7128), 361–365.

Internet

See: http://www.phru.nhs.uk/casp/rct.pdf

See: http://www.jr2.ox.ac.uk/bandolier/booth/booths/trials.html

See: http://www.clinicalevidence.com/ceweb/resources/index.jsp. You can use the Resources section of the site for useful materials and tools, including the EBM introductory workshop intended to help beginners with the following questions:

- What is EBM and how does it relate to me?
- What problems can it help me solve?
- What are the basic principles underlying EBM and how might I apply them to my own work?
- Where can I go for more information?

GIVING FEEDBACK

Feedback is given to colleagues, employers and students. In the exam, a question about giving an employee feedback on her performance at work tests the doctor's feedback technique. Doctors often use Pendleton's Rules to structure their feedback (see below).

WHAT IS GOOD FEEDBACK?

Feedback must enable change. Feedback is about telling people about specific aspects of their behaviour in a way that facilitates their adoption of more effective behaviours. These can be about their consulting behaviour or the way they interact with staff or the way in which they teach. It is about getting people to improve and also about motivating them so that they feel these improvements are not out of their reach. For feedback to do this, it needs to be:

- Specific: 'When you discussed the hospital referral with your patient, she looked surprised.' This is more specific than, 'Your consultation was awful. The poor woman left in tears.'
- Selective: Address one or two key issues rather than too many at once.
- Honest: Don't be dishonestly kind. Tackle ethical and attitudinal issues. 'When you spoke to the receptionist, you sounded patronising.' This is different to, 'You are patronising and sarcastic.' You have distinguished between the behaviour that needs changing and the personality of the individual. Keep feedback directed to behaviour that can be changed.
- Helpful: offer alternatives. 'I wonder if you had tried ...'; or 'Sometimes I find it helpful...' or 'Have you considered..' The person needs to identify and address the behaviour that needs changing.
- Sensitive: nobody likes to be told that their behaviour was lacking, and that changes are recommended. They respond by attacking the bearer of the news, or feeling deflated ('I tried my best and it still isn't good enough'), or by becoming defensive. Their effort needs to be acknowledged and appreciated so that they feel heard and understood. Only then will they feel motivated to continue.

Effective feedback requires a combination of qualities, skills and some structure. A person's performance is boosted by providing challenge with an appropriate level of support. The key skills are to listen and to ask, not to 'show and tell.'

WHY USE PENDLETON'S RULES?

Pendleton recognised that people have insight into their strengths and weaknesses. By allowing them to discuss their insights, you are harnessing their intrinsic motivation to improve. By discussing the positive aspects of their behaviour, you are acknowledging their effort and contribution. By then tackling the areas for improvement, you are identifying specific behaviours that need to change and suggesting ideas for improvement.

What are Pendleton's rules?

1. The recipients of the feedback go first and describe what went well and which of their strengths they demonstrated.
2. The person giving feedback goes next and also discusses their strengths. This acknowledges the other person's effort – it is encouraging. It also allays their anxiety.
3. The recipients then discuss how things may be done differently.
4. The person giving feedback then makes suggestions. For the suggestions to effect a change in behaviour, they have to be specific, honest, helpful and sensitive.

Advantages of Pendleton's rules

- With increasing familiarity, the rules provide a useful tool by which to structure feedback.
- The recipients are left with a clear summary of their strengths and an action plan for their improvement.
- Destructive criticism is minimised. The feedback concentrates on the person's behaviour and does not degenerate into an unhelpful attack on his personality.
- The recipients develop insight and a realistic understanding of the strengths and weaknesses of the performance.

Disadvantages of Pendleton's rules

- The feedback can be disjointed. People tend to remember events chronologically and may find it difficult to analyse the event in terms of 'things that went well' and 'areas for improvement'.
- The recipients and appraiser may disagree. If the parties disagree about the behaviour being a strength or a weakness, a confrontation develops. It is difficult to facilitate change in a confrontational environment.

Receiving feedback

- The recipient should listen to the feedback with an open mind and assume that it is constructive. However, it is difficult not to be defensive. The more time spent on convincing someone of the need to change, the less time available for discussing how to change.
- If the recipient did not understand what was said, he should ask for examples and clarify the advice. The person giving the feedback may be very experienced, or in a rush, or embarrassed and may say things quickly, using jargon. If the recipient wants to improve, he needs to understand exactly what needs changing and discuss ideas for improvement.
- The recipient should thank the person for their time and the thought they put into helping him develop.

LEARNING POINTS

Effective feedback requires a combination of:

- **qualities:** someone who is sensitive, honest, helpful, tactful and insightful
- **skills:** skills of communication – asking a balance of open, reflective, facilitating and closed questions; challenging and summarising
- **structure:** Pendleton's model

RELEVANT LITERATURE

King J (1999) **Giving feedback.** *BMJ Classified*, **26,** 2–3.
Parikh A, McReelis K, Hodges B (2001) **Student feedback in problem based learning: a survey of 103 final year students across five Ontario medical schools.** *Medical Education*, **35,** 632–36.
Ward D (2003) **Self-esteem and audit feedback.** *Nursing Standard*, **17,** 33–36.

REFLECTIVE LEARNING AND MENTORING

DEFINITION

Reflection is the process of deliberately and methodically considering past actions and learning lessons on what worked and what didn't and arriving at a plan of what to do next.

Reflective learning is seen as one of many tools for self-directed learning and development. The aim of reflective learning is for the doctor to develop self-awareness, to confirm his strengths and to identify his areas for improvement. As a result of developing self-awareness, the doctor's practice should improve.

TYPES OF REFLECTION

Reflection can be formal or informal; facilitated or self-conducted. In medicine, doctors are becoming increasingly familiar with mentorship or appraisal. Here the doctor's reflection is facilitated by a colleague. Formal facilitated reflection is a relatively new concept in medicine, whereas it is deeply embedded in nursing practice where it is called clinical supervision. There are many models of clinical supervision – Driscoll's '**What?**' model (2000) being one.

The framework of Driscoll's '**What?**' model comprises:

- '**What?**': A description of the events. What happened?
- '**So what?**': An analysis of the event. What resulted from these events? How did people feel?
- '**Now what?**': Proposed actions following the event. What can you do now and should this occur again, what can you do differently?

Driscoll's trigger questions are:

1. A description of the event: **What?**
   - What is the purpose of returning to the situation?
   - What happened?
   - What did I see / do?
   - What was my reaction to it?
   - What did other people that were involved in this do?
2. An analysis of the event: **So what?**
   - How did I feel at the time of the event?
   - Were those feelings I had any different from those of other people who were also involved at the time?
   - Are my feelings now, after the event, any different from those I experienced at the time?
   - Do I still feel troubled? If so, in what way?
   - What were the effects of what I did (or did not do)?

- What positive aspects emerge for me from the event?
- What have I noticed about my behaviour in practice by taking a more measured look at it?
- What observations does any person helping me to reflect on my practice make about the way I acted at the time?
3. Proposed actions following the event: **Now what?**
   - What are the implications for me and others in clinical practice based on what I have described and analysed?
   - What difference does it make if I choose to do nothing?
   - Where can I get more information to face a similar situation again?
   - How can I modify my practice if a similar situation were to happen again?
   - What help do I need to help me 'action' the results of my reflections?
   - Which aspect should be tackled first?
   - How will I notice that I am any different in clinical practice?
   - What is the main learning that I take from reflecting on my practice in this way?

THE BENEFITS OF FACILITATED REFLECTION

The facilitator provides a supportive, non-judgemental environment. However, within this supportive climate, challenging questions are asked. Challenging the doctor within a supportive environment is ideal for a doctor's growth and development – challenge without support is seen as an attack whereas support with no challenge is seen as molly coddling.

A facilitator does not say, 'You are bad at explaining things to patients!' A facilitator will ask the doctor questions: 'Why did your patient became angry? Could you do it differently next time? How would you do it differently?' By asking these questions, the doctor will hopefully become aware of his deficiencies and will hence gain insight into the problem. Hopefully he will correct the problem without the facilitator's prompting and will be more insightful of his behaviours in the future.

Facilitated reflection is useful for exposing blind spots – see *Figure 2*. Johari's window is a pictorial representation of the facilitator's knowledge (Y axis) and doctor's knowledge (X axis). The aim of facilitated reflection is to reduce the 'blind-spot' by the facilitator 'feeding back' what he knows about the doctor to him. The facilitator challenges the doctor's deeply held assumptions (his blind-spots) and encourages him to question the validity of these assumptions. By making the doctor overtly conscious of his assumptions, the doctor becomes aware of how others perceive him. This increased self-awareness can be directed towards making effective adaptations to his behaviour.

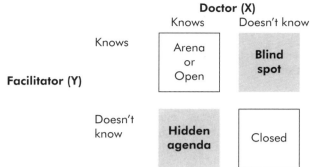

Figure 2. Johari's window

MENTORING IN GENERAL PRACTICE

Mentoring is defined as:

'an experienced highly regarded empathic person (the mentor) guides another individual (the mentee) in the development and re-examination of his or her own ideas, learning, personal, and professional developments. This is achieved by listening and talking in confidence.'

Standing Committee on Postgraduate Medical and Dental Education (1999)

Responsibilities of mentor and mentee

Mentors facilitate the process of constructive reflection. The mentees set the agenda – they determine the topics or incidents they wish to reflect upon. The meeting usually takes place at the surgery – the content of the meeting is often confidential, making public venues unsuitable (Alliot, 1996). Meetings usually last between 60 and 90 minutes. For mentoring to be successful, a caring and trusting relationship must develop between mentor and mentee.

Grainger (2002) identified the three most common instances when people find the mentorship useful:

- Mentees who are new to an organisation.
- Mentees who are concerned with their career development.
- Mentees who are being developed for future leadership positions.

MENTORING DOS AND DON'TS

Adapted from Grainger (2002).

Dos

- Listen carefully and watch for non-verbal cues
- Facilitate the mentee's development – do not expect your mentee to do what you would do
- Help with networking
- Be honest with feedback – be direct, constructive, and kind when making suggestions

- Maintain confidentiality
- Make notes if these help maintain the focus of your discussions from one meeting to the next
- Discuss in advance with your mentee what the two of you would do in emotionally stressful discussions – safety net

Don'ts
- Don't shy away from giving 'negative' feedback, but avoid being unnecessarily critical. Describe the behaviour, not the personality.
- Don't abuse your authority as a mentor. Recognise that a power differential exists.
- Don't expect your mentee to defer to you.
- Don't use your mentee's achievements to further your own agenda.

CUED MODELLING

Cued modelling is a process of highlighting examples of good practice. It is the result of deliberate analysis by the facilitator and the doctor – what was it that made a particular behaviour successful or less successful? How did the doctor feel when this behaviour occurred and why? The motivations and consequences of the doctor's actions are discussed to develop awareness of his own behaviours. For example, a doctor may pick up that a patient is depressed and based on his intuition, he may sensitively probe the issue. The facilitator, in analysing this piece of behaviour, asks the doctor how he picked up the depressive symptoms and why he chose the questions he used. The doctor then becomes consciously aware of his good consulting behaviours – his ability to use his intuition, his ability to time his questions well and to use silence to allow the patient space in which to explore her feelings. In facilitation, the doctor develops self-awareness – he gains insight into his good (and less good) consulting techniques.

UNCONDITIONED POSITIVE REGARD

Facilitators need to be sensitive to the effort that the doctor has put into his work and to value his contribution before attempting to address his deficiencies. Rogers (1983) called this 'unconditioned positive regard'. If a warm and understanding atmosphere is created, then deficits in knowledge, attitudes and skills may be explored without these being interpreted as a negative comment on the doctor personally. Balanced feedback is important: the doctor must come to an understanding of what he needs to improve but he must leave feeling motivated to make these changes.

ROLE PLAY

In facilitated reflection, role play can be used to try out new ways of doing things. A doctor may role play a situation to gain a greater understanding of the dynamics.

ADDITIONAL INFORMATION

ROGER (Reciprocal Observation, Guidance, Education, and Reflection) is a newly developed teaching tool that offers opportunities for reflection (Williams P and Bache J, 2004).

The ROGER process has five essential elements:

- It is a *Reciprocal* process. One professional acts as the appraiser and the other acts as the appraisee. They then reverse roles and repeat the process.
- *Observation* of the normal practice of the appraisee is undertaken by the appraiser, normally without interruption.
- The appraiser then offers *Guidance* to the appraisee. This guidance may be clinical or related to other aspects of the consultation—for example, communication skills.
- An opportunity exists for *Education* through observation of good practice, feedback on the consultation, and discussion of clinical topics. Education is usually clinical – for example, interpretation of electrocardiograms, radiological interpretation, pharmacological options, management options.
- Finally, there is opportunity for *Reflection*. What was done well? Could the consultation have been improved? Was treatment appropriate? Could communication have been better? What was learnt today?

RELEVANT LITERATURE

Alliott R (1996) **Facilitating mentoring in general practice.** *BMJ, Career Focus,* **313**(7060).

Butterworth T et al. (2001) **Clinical supervision and mentorship in nursing.** *Stanley Thornes Ltd,* Cheltenham.

Casement P (1985) **On learning from the patient.** *Routledge,* London.

Cottrell D et al. (2002) **What is effective supervision and how does it happen? A critical incident study.** *Medical Education,* **36,** 1042–1049.

Cowan L (2000) Lessons from experience: working with students in community midwifery practice. In: Spouse J and Redfern L (eds) **Successful supervision in health care practice.** *Blackwell Science Ltd.,* Oxford, pp. 50–57.

Driscoll J (2000) **Practising clinical supervision: A reflective approach.** *Balliere Tindall,* Edinburgh.

Grainger C (2002) **Mentoring: supporting doctors at work and at play.** *BMJ,* **324,** S203.

Grant J et al. (1999) **The good CPD guide.** Reed Healthcare Publishing, Sutton.

Havelock P et al. (1995) **Professional education for general practice.** Oxford University Press, Oxford.

Rogers, C. (1983) **Freedom to learn for the 80s.** Merrill Macmillan Publishing Co., New York.

Wilkinson TJ et al. 2002. **The use of portfolios for assessment for practice of the competence and performance of doctors in practice.** Medical Education, **36,** 918–924.

Williams P and Bache J (2004) **Learning with ROGER.** BMJ Career Focus, **329,** 58–59.

Winstanley J and White E (2003) **Clinical supervision: models, measures and best practice.** Nurse Researcher, **10**(4), 7–38.

Van Zwanenberg T and Harrison J (eds) (2003) **Clinical governance for primary care.** Radcliffe Medical Press, Oxon.

MANAGING CHANGE

Questions on managing change appear in many guises, such as:

- How would you set up a patient participation group in your practice?
- What is your practice's strategy for achieving 48 hour access for patients?
- Your partner wishes to introduce a practice counsellor. What are the issues?
- Your practice wishes to develop a website. Discuss potential options.
- Your partner wants the practice to become more involved in research. What would you need to consider?

Just as there are models for breaking bad news, negotiating a difficult consultation or giving feedback, there are models for managing change. A comprehensive discussion of all the change models is beyond this chapter. The following models will be discussed:

- Model for Improvement
- RAID model
- Kaufman's discrepancy model
- Lewin's force-field analysis

MODEL FOR IMPROVEMENT

The NHS Modernisation Agency uses the Model for Improvement. Its framework includes:

- **Asking three key questions**
  What are we trying to accomplish?
  How will we know that a change is an improvement?
  What changes can we make that will result in improvement?

- **It uses a process for testing change ideas:** Plan, Do, Study, Act (PDSA) cycles.

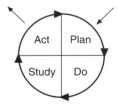

The PDSA cycle:
- Plan: plan the change to be tested or implemented
- Do: carry out the test or change
- Study: study data before and after the change and reflect on what was learnt
- Act: plan the next change cycle or plan implementation

FEATURES OF THE MODEL FOR IMPROVEMENT

- Ideas are tested on a small scale first
  - Less disruptive to employees / patients
  - Each cycle builds on the previous learning – incremental, structured, less threatening change occurs
  - Different people are involved in many small changes – higher chance of success
- Small changes involve less time, money and risk
- Some changes do not work – people learn from these before new changes are made
- The ideas and changes are 'owned' by the team – there is less resistance to change

RAID MODEL

RAID is the model for change currently used by the Clinical Governance Support Team of the Modernisation Agency. RAID stands for:

- Review: look at the current situation and prepare the organisation for change
- Agree: ensure staff are signed up to the proposed changes
- Implement: put in place the proposed changes
- Demonstrate: show that the changes have made improvements

KAUFMAN'S DISCREPANCY MODEL

- Where are we now? To answer this question, identify what we have and what we lack, i.e. do a needs analysis, using a SWOT analysis or a Manchester rating scale.
- Where do we want to get to? These outcomes must be SMART (specific, measurable, achievable, realistic, time-bound).

LEWIN'S FORCE-FIELD ANALYSIS

- Where are we now?
- Where do we want to be?
- What are factors resisting change?
- What are the drivers encouraging change?

This model recognises that change is achieved by tackling the resisting factors. If the drivers are increased in the face of opposition, resistance simply increases. For change to occur, the resisting factors should be reduced.

DEVELOPING A LEARNING ORGANISATION

Managing change locally (at practice level) and managing change more widely (at PCT and NHS level) have many things in common – the same change management models can be used. In addition, the correct organisational culture needs to be developed. An organisation that fosters a culture that supports learning is called a 'learning organisation.' Learning organisations create an atmosphere of sharing their experience to keep up with changes; these organisations do not reinvent the wheel.

Peter Senge, a professor of management, wrote about the five disciplines of a learning organisation. These are: systems thinking, personal mastery, mental models, shared vision, and team learning.

- Systems thinking: See the whole picture and recognise the patterns and interactions within the system. Success depends on reinforcing or changing the underlying patterns, not just completing a series of tasks.
- Personal mastery: Three important elements are personal vision, creative tension and commitment to truth.
    - Personal vision: This is about what you want (your goal) and why you want it (your purpose).
    - Creative tension: There are unavoidable gaps between one's vision and current reality. Gaps are a source of creative energy. There are only two ways to resolve the tension between reality and the vision. Either vision pulls reality toward it, or reality pulls vision downward.
    - Commitment to truth: Be honest about the limiting factors. The underlying structures need to be changed to produce results.
- Mental models: Our understanding of the world is based on our assumptions. New ideas rarely get put into practice because they conflict with deeply held assumptions. To improve, current mental models must be questioned and challenged.
- Shared vision: Everybody within the organisation needs to have a clear idea of what they want to create – shared visions create focus and energy. They give a sense of purpose and coherence to all the activities the organisation carries out.
- Team learning: Each member is committed and shares a vision of greatness. The team's collective competence is far greater than any individual's.

LEARNING POINTS

- Model for Improvement; RAID model; Kaufman's discrepancy model; Lewin's force-field analysis
- Plan, Do, Study, Act (PDSA) cycles
- For change to occur, the resisting factors (obstacles) should be reduced.
- Senge – the five disciplines of a learning organisation

ADDITIONAL INFORMATION

Consider the move away from PGEA to PDPs – this was an organisational change in the funding and delivery of continuing professional development to GPs.

The old system of GP education was based on PGEA.

Criticisms levelled at PGEA:

- the top-down didactic approach (mainly lecture-based)
- its non-inclusiveness (addressed the talkers' interests and rarely considered the learners' learning needs)
- not involving learners (in what, how and when the learning was delivered)
- failing to influence working behaviour (education was responsible for only one third of the changes seen in clinical practice)
- has been open to abuse and yielded little professional satisfaction – 'bums on seats'.

What was the vision for GP education?

The vision was to provide an effective education that met the needs of the patient, the NHS and the practitioner, including GPs with special interests. Educationalists wanted a more 'adult-learning' orientated system. The GMC wanted a system that met the requirements for appraisal and revalidation.

How was this new vision going to be delivered?

The Chief Medical Officer (Calman, 1998) advocated the use of Personal Development Plans (PDPs). Drivers for change included the drive for multi-professional education, inter-professional education and the focus on outcome-based education (results-orientated thinking). A credit based system of education (as used in Australia and South Africa) could have been introduced, however reviews evaluating credit based educational schemes show that these do not lead to changes in behaviour or organisational improvements.

It was proposed that PDPs would bring medical education into the realms of adult education principles. However, PDPs have met with great resistance, with pressure of work and lack of protected time being quoted as reasons for resisting uptake. Also the introduction of PDPs is seen as being a top-down process. Despite these arguments, PDPs were introduced.

The system will need evaluation. What outcomes do we evaluate? It is not the provision of educational opportunities which improves patient care, it is the reflection and application of the learning. Therefore outcomes to be measured need to show the effectiveness of the education – changes in practice not numbers of doctors participating.

The change in GP education can be reviewed as:

- Plan: change from PGEA
- Do: set up a new system. Reject credit based education in favour of PDPs
- Study: reflect on whether these changes have delivered our vision (evaluate)
- Act: make changes to the PDP system to make the process more robust, or change to a new system.

Did the NHS use Senge's principles:

- Systems thinking: Yes. The entire system of funding, organising and delivering GP education changed.
- Personal mastery: PDPs were a top-down approach – educationalists wanted it; the GMC revalidation procedures needed it; the Government's agenda in *A first class service* liked it. There wasn't much of a shared vision amongst grass-roots GPs.
- Mental models: The model of education as 'chalk and talk' was questioned and replaced by a model of adult education or 'learner-centred learning.'
- Shared vision: Not really!
- Team learning: Once the system was introduced, ideas on PDPs were shared in the medical literature and by the local deaneries.

RELEVANT LITERATURE

Calman K. (1998). **A review of continuing professional development in general practice.** DoH, London. http://open.gov.uk/doh/cme/cmoh.htm
Davies HTO and Nutley SM (2000) **Developing learning organizations in the new NHS.** *BMJ*, **320,** 998–1001.
http://www.modern.nhs.uk/improvementguides/patients/
http://www.modern.nhs.uk/improvementguides/process/2_4.html
http://www.jr2.ox.ac.uk/bandolier/ImpAct/imp01/BACKPAGE.html
http://www.nelh.nhs.uk/folio/mchip/future_developments.htm
http://www.infed.org/thinkers/senge.htm

ETHICAL FRAMEWORKS

Doctors are most familiar with the four ethical principles of:

- **Autonomy:** People of sound mind should have the right to determine what happens to them (literally, self-rule). Respect for patient autonomy requires doctors to help patients come to their own decisions, for example by providing important information in a way they can understand. Doctors should respect their patients and follow their decisions even when they believe that the patient is wrong. The doctor has a duty to respect the rights and dignity of the person, to promote their well-being, and to be truthful, honest and sincere.
- **Beneficence:** Doctors should do good and promote what is best for their patients. The principle of autonomy captures the patient's views; the principle of beneficence captures the doctors' views of the patient's best interests. The two principles conflict when competent patients choose a course of action that is not in their best interests (Piccoli *et al.*, 2004). The doctor has a duty to inform and educate the person, enhancing his capability to continue care for himself.
- **Non-maleficence:** First do no harm. The potential good and harm of a therapeutic intervention need to be weighed up to decide what, overall, is in the patient's best interests.
- **Justice:** When doctors make decisions, their actions should be fair not only to the patient, but also to others. Doctors must try to distribute limited resources (time, money, expensive treatments) fairly. The doctor has a duty to avoid discrimination, abuse or exploitation of people on grounds of race, age, class, gender or religion.

WHY ARE ETHICAL THEORIES IMPORTANT?

Ethical theories can help you to consider various aspects of a situation so that you can weigh up the pros and cons of each course of action. Ethical theories don't tell you which course of action to follow. Different people have different values, so their actions will be different, but they may need to justify why they have chosen a particular course of action. Ethical theories provide the basis for justifying specific ethical decisions.

Consider the following scenario. You go Christmas shopping with your teenage niece. She chooses a bright orange and purple coat. She smiles excitedly and says to you, 'Does this look cool?' You are faced with a moral dilemma. You can take a step back and apply a few ethical frameworks to the dilemma to weigh up the pros and cons of each possible course of action.

ETHICAL THEORIES

Three ethical theories can be applied to the above scenario:

- **Duty based ethics** (deontology) – These state that an action is right if it is in accord with a moral rule or principle. Certain acts are wrong in themselves, independent of their foreseeable consequences.

  With regard to the scenario, lying is wrong, so you should tell your niece the truth irrespective of the hurt you cause.

  Deontology impacts on how we practise as doctors. The GMC produced *The duties of a doctor* – a code of practice that considers the doctors' duties and the patients' rights. Beneficence (doing good) and non-maleficence (not doing harm) are principally about the duty that doctors have to patients.

- **Utilitarianism ethics, particularly consequentialism** – These principles state that an action is right if it promotes the best consequences – the greatest good or happiness for the greatest number. Those actions that promote, or intend to promote, more happiness are better than those that promote less happiness. A weakness of this theory is that it is not possible to measure happiness.

  With regard to the scenario, lying to your niece now may make her happy, but on your return home, her mother may be unhappy with the choice of coat and disallow its wearing. Your niece would be unhappy and so would you for being instrumental in the conflict.

- **Virtue ethics** – These state that an action is right if it is what a virtuous agent would do in the circumstances. The central focus is the moral character of the person, e.g. kind, generous, and empathetic. A weakness of this theory is that it is tied to cultural norms – a virtuous doctor half a century ago may have been one who was paternalistic with little consideration for patient autonomy.

  With regard to the scenario, you could spend a bit more time looking and find a present that pleases both of you and would have the approval of her mother. You would be generous with your time, considerate of your niece's (and her mother's) feelings.

THE LAW

Consent is the expression, in law, of the ethical principle of autonomy. In seeking consent from a patient, a doctor has the duty to ensure that:

1. The consenting patient has capacity.
2. The consenting patient is appropriately informed before making a decision.
3. The consent is given voluntarily.

Patients are presumed **competent** unless they are shown to lack decision-making capacity.

The current test of competence was set by Judge J. Thorpe in the case known as Re C.

To meet the test of competence, the patient must:

1. comprehend and retain the necessary information,
2. believe it,
3. weigh the information, balancing risks and needs, to arrive at a true choice.

The law differs slightly in its treatment of adults and minors.

LEARNING POINTS

- Deontology, utilitarianism and virtue ethics
- Consent
- Competence

ADDITIONAL INFORMATION

The treatment of an adult
The treatment of the adult depends on whether she is competent, or not.

- If the adult is incompetent, she can be treated in her best interests.
- If the adult is competent, she has the right to refuse medical treatment, even if the treatment is life-saving or life-sustaining.

But a patient, competent or incompetent, can be detained under sections 2 or 3 of the Mental Health Act (MHA) 1983 if she meets the criteria for detention. If she is detained, even if she is competent, she can be treated without her consent, under section 63 of the MHA 1983.

The treatment of a minor
A minor aged sixteen or seventeen can be treated in the same way as an adult, and competence assessed using the adult test of competence.

If the patient is *under the age of sixteen*, competence will be tested using the Fraser guidelines. Judge Fraser formulated these guidelines in the Gillick case. Consent for treatment may be obtained from a minor if:

- The implications of the treatment are understood
- Seeking of parental advice is encouraged
- Without treatment, the minor is still likely to pursue the course of action
- The minor's health needs and best interests are met by giving the treatment.

Therefore, a Gillick competent child may give consent to medical treatment, although refusal of consent may be overridden.

The GMC guidance in assessing the patient's best interests
In deciding what options may be reasonably considered as being in the best interests of a patient who lacks capacity to decide, you should take into account:

- options for treatment or investigation which are clinically indicated;
- any evidence of the patient's previously expressed preferences, including an advance statement; your own and the health care team's knowledge of the patient's background, such as cultural, religious, or employment considerations;
- views about the patient's preferences given by a third party who may have other knowledge of the patient, for example the patient's partner, family, carer, tutor-dative (Scotland), or a person with parental responsibility;
- which option least restricts the patient's future choices, where more than one option (including non-treatment) seems reasonable in the patient's best interest.

There are conditions which must be satisfied under section 63 of the Mental Health Act before the patient can be treated:

1. The patient must be detained under the Act.
2. The treatment proposed must count as 'medical treatment'.
3. The treatment proposed must constitute treatment for the mental disorder.

If the detained patient is competent, it is best practice to obtain her consent to treatment. If she does not consent, the doctor may proceed with treatment in the patient's best interests, as is therapeutically necessary. If the patient resists the treatment, the doctor can use such restraint as is clinically necessary.

RELEVANT LITERATURE

Journal articles

Greenhallgh T, Kostopoulou O, and Harries C (2004) **Making decisions about benefits and harms of medicines.** *BMJ*, **329**, 47–50.
Parker MJ (2004) **Getting ethics into practice.** *BMJ*, **329**, 126.
Piccoli GB, Mezza E, Grassi G, Burdese M, and Todros T (2004) **Interactice case report. A 35 year old woman with diabetic nephropathy who wants a baby: case outcome.** *BMJ*, **329**, 900–903.
Pollard JP and Savullescu J (2004) **Ethics in practice: eligibility of overseas visitors and people of uncertain residential status for NHS treatment.** *BMJ*, **329**, 346–349.

Books

Orme-Smith A, Spicer J **Ethics in General Practice.** *Radcliffe Medical Press*, Oxon.
Kennedy I, Grubb A (2000) **Medical Law,** 3rd edition. *Butterworths*, Oxford.

Internet

http://www.gmc-uk.org/global_sections/search_frameset.htm
http://www.gmc-uk.org/standards/default.htm

PROFESSIONALISM

Why do I need to know about professionalism for the MRCGP exam?
Professionalism can be incorporated into any question. The oral exam tests the doctors' professional values and professional growth. A question on professional values may appear in many guises, such as:

- Do you think that doctors should participate in appraisal and revalidation?
- How would you deal with an ill partner?

WHY IS PROFESSIONALISM IMPORTANT IN GENERAL PRACTICE?

- As doctors we are expected to follow a code of ethics. The public have certain expectations of us and we have certain responsibilities to them.
- Since the introduction of appraisal and revalidation, doctors are expected to demonstrate evidence of their professional development.

The doctors' code of ethics incorporates the attitudes, values and beliefs that the profession and the public have agreed on. These are stated in the GMC's *Good medical practice* as:

- make the care of your patient your first concern;
- treat every patient politely and considerately;
- respect patients' dignity and privacy;
- listen to patients and respect their views;
- give patients information in a way they can understand;
- respect the rights of patients to be fully involved in decisions about their care;
- keep your professional knowledge and skills up to date;
- recognise the limits of your professional competence;
- be honest and trustworthy;
- respect and protect confidential information;
- make sure that your personal beliefs do not prejudice your patients' care;
- act quickly to protect patients from risk if you have good reason to believe that you or a colleague may not be fit to practise;
- avoid abusing your position as a doctor; and
- work with colleagues in the ways that best serve patients' interests.

In all these matters doctors must never discriminate unfairly against their patients or colleagues and they must always be prepared to justify their actions to them.

CHARACTERISTICS OF PROFESSIONALISM

Central to the concept of professionalism are four attributes:

1. **Putting patients' interests first** – Rationing and payment for medical treatment may conflict with this principle.

2. **Ethical behaviour** – doctors should not breach confidence or take advantage of their position or abuse drugs to which they have access.
3. **Being responsive to society** – doctors need to adapt to a changing society e.g. a move away from the paternalism of the 1950s to increased patient choice and a respect for patients' autonomy.
4. **Being humane** – behaving with empathy, integrity, altruism and trustworthiness.

(Swick, 1999)

WHAT DEFINES THE MEDICAL PROFESSION?

1. The medical profession holds specialised knowledge and is responsible for imparting this knowledge to its students.
2. This knowledge is used to improve the lives of patients.
3. The profession is self-regulating. It establishes and maintains its own standards of practice.
4. The profession is responsible for its research.

The contract with society was renegotiated recently following several high profile scandals (Shipman, Alder Hay and Bristol). Following the Bristol scandal, there was a confidential inquiry which highlighted deficiencies in the professional conduct of some doctors. The GMC heeded these recommendations and changed its licensing procedures accordingly. If these changes had not been made, the profession was in danger of losing its self-regulatory powers. These changes have been called 'New Professionalism'.

LEARNING POINTS

- Doctors' code of ethics and professionalism – GMC's *Good medical practice*
- The four attributes of professionalism (Swick, 1999)
- 'New Professionalism' (Stacey, 1992)
- Bristol Royal Infirmary Inquiry (1996) highlighted the cultural changes that need to occur to improve the professionalism of doctors
- Emphasis on greater lay involvement, peer appraisal, accountability, quality assurance and transparency within the NHS

ADDITIONAL INFORMATION

The Bristol Royal Infirmary Inquiry
In 1996 parents of children undergoing routine cardiac operations wrote to the GMC asking for an investigation into the practice of three doctors (Mr Dhasmana who had 20 deaths following 38 arterial switch operations; Mr Wisheart who had 9 deaths following 15 atrio-ventricular septal defect operations;

and Dr Roylance who was the chief executive of the United Bristol Healthcare NHS Trust).

After a consultant anaesthetist reported his concerns, an independent review investigated. In 1998, the GMC found all three doctors guilty of serious professional misconduct. In a landmark decision, Dr Roylance, in his administrative, not clinical capacity, was found guilty due to his failure to *act upon concerns*. This was seen as an act of collusion with poorly performing doctors at the expense of society.

In June 1998, Professor Ian Kennedy, a law professor, was appointed to conduct an inquiry. The aim of the inquiry, the biggest in the history of the NHS, was to uncover all aspects of what went wrong.

The King's Fund report summarised the findings and recommendations of the inquiry as follows:

Events similar to Bristol are unlikely to happen again for three reasons:

- Professional bodies and NHS managers will regularly audit outcomes of treatment and will need to explain variations in performance against peers.
- The attitude and accountability of professionals is undergoing change, and it is now a professional requirement to report concerns about the performance of colleagues – 'whistleblowing'.
- The public and media are holding the health service to account, and asking for data on performance measures, such as league tables.

Changes to the culture that allowed the events at Bristol to happen, have occurred:

- There is greater public involvement in professional regulation.
- A formal process of local, peer appraisal and regular GMC revalidation has been rolled out.
- There are attempts to change the culture of the NHS to a more open, less blaming culture. Cultural change is recognised as a difficult task.

The public expressed concerns with the following aspects of medical professionalism:

1. Deficiencies in self-regulation and quality of care

(i) The public felt that the medical profession turned a blind eye to poorly performing doctors who potentially harmed patients.

'Medicine has been excessively paternalistic, too tolerant of poor practice, and lacking in openness about clinical ability.'   (Irvine, 2001)

But in attempting to maintain its self-regulation, the pendulum may have swung too far.

'..the arm of self-regulation in medicine can be seen as attempting to convince those concerned that registration represents more than competence and professional probity but a conscience beyond reproach; a superhuman paragon of virtue'.

Such was Case's (2003) comment in her legal analysis of GMC hearings following the 1995 reforms. She goes even further:

'protecting the dignity of the profession is borne out of self interest and therefore might undermine the GMC's efforts to protect the broader public interest'.

(ii) With the move away from individual doctoring to team doctoring, a blame culture needs to be replaced by a culture of openness and a willingness to acknowledge and learn from our mistakes.

In trying to develop a blame-free, responsible and robust culture, Liam Donaldson proposed a systems approach to error. This involves looking at the technical, organisational, social, and communication factors that predispose to human error.

'The recognition that human error is inevitable in a highly complex and technical field like medicine is a first step in promoting greater self awareness of the importance of systems failure in the causation of accidents.'

(Donaldson, 2002)

2. Conflict between the doctor's advocacy role and his gatekeeper role

The doctor is the patient's advocate. He needs to put his patients' interests first. However, he has a duty to distribute limited healthcare resources efficiently. For example, a doctor may want to prescribe beta-interferon to his multiple sclerosis patients, but if all doctors did this, the health service would soon be bankrupted! His relationship with the patient is strained by his duty to the wider public.

Due to this increasing conflict, NICE was established in April 1999. NICE reviews the evidence with regard to the cost-effectiveness and clinical effectiveness of new and existing therapies with a view to issuing guidelines to the NHS. Some people argue that NICE is a rationing organisation. However, NICE's advice still puts doctors in difficult positions with the patient. As in the above example of MS, NICE does not recommend the use of beta-interferon on the grounds that it is neither curative nor cost-effective. The doctor knows that beta-interferon will help to reduce the debilitating symptoms experienced by MS sufferers, and in not prescribing it he is not acting in the patient's best interests.

3. Less altruistic behaviour on the part of some doctors

There are concerns about poorly performing doctors and the tendency of the profession to close ranks. The GMC needs to be seen as an organisation that polices its doctors. The GMC needs to identify and deal with the poorly performing doctors. In response, revalidation has been developed. However, there is scepticism that revalidation will successfully identify poor performance and poor professionalism – those who need revalidation most are unlikely to be recognised by this system. Would it have identified Harold Shipman?

The GMC's response: New professionalism

'New professionalism' was a term coined by Stacey (1992) to describe the qualities of good doctoring that the public and the medical profession together agree upon and the means of delivering them effectively. The Bristol inquiry spurred on the GMC reforms and

> 'resulted in the construction of a new government framework for the regulation of medicine, putting the safety of patients treated by the NHS first... However good the systems and institutions are that govern medicine, they will only work properly if doctors are clinically competent, honest, and want to provide a consistently good standard of practice and care.' (Irvine, 2001)

And so revalidation was born. Irvine recognised that changing the rules, structures and processes was easy; changing the attitudes of the medical profession would be far more difficult. New professionalism was the key to change.

The early changes were:

- Public involvement in medical regulation increased, with the doubling of the lay proportion on the Privy Council between 1995 and 2000.
- The GMC was restructured into a more proactive, quality-orientated organisation, assuring clinicians' fitness to practise.
- '*Good medical practice* is an explicit statement of duties, responsibilities, values, and standards for doctors, based on a strong public and professional consensus about the qualities that are important' (Irvine, 2001). The new standards for the profession were agreed, explicitly stated and policed.
- Compliance with the principles of *Good medical practice* will be secured by the changes to the medical curriculum, and by revalidation. Doctors who breach *Good medical practice* will be supported until they reach an acceptable level of practice.

> 'To ensure patient safety, the new professionalism requires professional leadership with greater public input to medical regulation, a modern GMC, and a closer fit between the licensure of doctors and the quality assurance of the organisations in which they work.' (Irvine, 2001)

The King's Fund has published a report – *On being a doctor: redefining medical professionalism* – which argues that while individual doctors remain highly trusted, confidence in the profession as a whole is being undermined. It highlights challenges, including growing public expectations of health care and government demands for more responsive public services.

RELEVANT LITERATURE

Case P (2003) **Confidence matters: the rise and fall of informational autonomy in medical law.** *Medical Law Review*, **11**, 208–29.

Cruess RL *et al.* (1999) **Renewing professionalism: an opportunity for medicine,** *Acad Med*, **74**, 878–84.

Cruess RL *et al.* (2000) **Professionalism: an ideal to be sustained.** *Lancet*, **356**, 156–59.

Donaldson L (2002) **An organisation with a memory.** *Clinical Medicine*, **2**, 452–57.

Epstein RM and Hundert EM (2002) **Defining and assessing professional competence.** *JAMA,* **287,** 226–35.

Horton R (2002) **The doctor's role in advocacy.** *The Lancet,* **359,** 458.

Hunter DJ (2000) **Managing the NHS.** *Health Care UK,* 69–76.

Irvine D (2001) **Doctors in the UK: their professionalism and its regulatory framework.** *The Lancet,* **58,** 1807–10.

Kennedy I, Grubb A (2000) **Medical Law.** 3rd edition. *Butterworths,* Oxford

King's Fund background briefing to the Bristol Royal Infirmary Inquiry (2003) King's Fund, London.

Neuberger J (2001) **The educated patient: new challenges for the medical profession.** *Journal of Internal Medicine,* **249,** 41–5.

Sculpher *et al.* (2002) **Shared treatment decision making in a collectively funded health care system: possible conflicts and some potential solutions.** *Social Science and Medicine,* **54,** 1369–77.

Smith R (2001) **Why are doctors so unhappy?** *BMJ,* **322,** 1073–4.

Spencer J (2003) **Teaching about professionalism.** *Medical Education,* **37,** 288–9.

Stacey M (1992) **Regulating British medicine: the General Medical Council.** *Wiley,* Chichester.

Swick HL *et al.* (1999) **Teaching professionalism in undergraduate medical education.** *JAMA,* **282,** 830–2.

MOCK QUESTIONS FOR EXAM PREPARATION

These can be done individually or in groups.

1. Are GPs affected by politics in medicine?
2. Do you think that patients, given the chance, would have voted positively for the new GMS contract?
3. Do you think that the new GMS contract will provide better patient-centred care?
4. One of the attributes of a good GP is the ability to deal with 'uncertainty' well. How do you deal with uncertainty? How do you know if you are dealing with uncertainty well?
5. A final year law student is sitting his exam tomorrow. He asks for antibiotics for a sore throat. What factors help you decide if you give them?
6. How would you react (as a locum doctor) to a request for a prescription for diazepam?
7. What would you do if you received a telephone result from the laboratory that a patient's potassium was 6.7? You are unable to get in touch with the patient.
8. A local GP is your patient. She requests a prescription for a slimming drug that she has read about in a diabetic journal. She meets the criteria for the drug but as it is so new, you have no experience of it. How would you react?
9. A mother phones you at the practice demanding a visit for her 9 year old child. What issues does this raise?
10. You do a home visit to see a 2 month old child who has been very sleepy. You find the child has a single mum who is drunk at your visit. How would you tackle this?
11. Would you prescribe to colleagues? What issues does this raise?
12. A mother asks you to write a letter to the Council to support her application for a larger flat. Her 16 year son has behavioural problems. What issues does this raise?
13. You attend the relatives of a patient who has just died whilst the carer had 'just popped to the shops'. The relatives ask you, 'What do we do Doctor?' How would you advise them?
14. GPs are encountered to have teenage-friendly practices. What does this mean and what issues does this raise?
15. A woman requests that you do not put her history of having had a termination of pregnancy on her insurance form. What issues does this raise?
16. Your colleague thinks you need a mentor – what issues does this raise?
17. How do you learn? How do you prioritise learning?
18. You get £5000 from the PCT for education – how would you use it?
19. Do you think lay people should sit on the Revalidation Committee for doctors?
20. How would you recognise a dysfunctional consultation, and what would you do about it?

21. The receptionists report that one of your patients is aggressive to them but this has not been your experience – the patient has always been nice to you. How do you deal with this?

22. Discuss the issues raised by having the practice manager as a profit-sharing partner.

23. A drug-rep offers to lend you the services of a specialist nurse to audit your asthma patients. What issues does this raise?

24. Does every general practice need a good leader? What happens if there are two leaders within the partnership?

25. Do you think that mentoring/appraisal should be conducted by people who are trained to do the job? Do you think that a doctor who is trained in communicating with patients has readily transferable skills? Do you think that mentoring/appraisal should be quality assured?

26. What isues does setting up a patient participation group for the surgery raise?

27. The local radio station invites you to participate in a Sunday session on teenage health issues. What issues does this raise? If you decide to participate, what communication skills would you employ?

28. What do you think are the differences between an underperforming doctor and a burnt out doctor? The PCT asks the trainer in your practice to 'supervise' an underperforming doctor. What issues does this raise?

29. How could you learn from your heartsink patients?

30. What are the advantages and disadvantages of telephone consultations?

31. The pharmacists within your PCT currently prescribe emergency contraception under patient group directives. Do you think that they should be trained in consultation skills? Which consultation model would you advocate and why?

32. How would you deal with a patient who presents with a list of problems?

33. Would you see representatives from the pharmaceutical industry? Discuss.

34. The PACT data shows that your senior partner has the largest expenditure within the PCT. What factors may influence this? What issues does it raise?

35. Do you think that pregnant women should be routinely asked about domestic violence?

36. A mother of Amy, a 6 year old insulin diabetic, admits to 'smacking' her daughter when Amy refused to have her supper after taking her insulin. What issues does this raise?

37. A father asks you for your advice on genetic testing. He believes that his 12 year old daughter may not be his child. What issues does this raise?

38. One of your partners consults quickly and sees most of the extra patients. A patient satisfaction survey showed that he is very popular. However, he does not complete the templates and this has resulted in fewer Quality and Outcome points. What issues does this raise?

39. Your practice nurse felt that the appraisal she had with the senior partner was rushed and inadequate. She requests that you do another appraisal. What issues does this raise?

40. One of your patients informs you that he was advised by the local homeopath to refuse his influenza vaccination. He is the fifth patient to volunteer this information. What issues does this raise?

INDEX

PUNS and DENs, 29, 38, 40

Reflective learning, 45, 165
Removal from list, 113

Screening, 64
   cervical cancer, 68
   chlamydia, 64
   Wilson's criteria, 64
Sick notes, 120

Significant event analysis, 31, 49, 110,
   155
SMART objectives, 107
Stress, 98

Utilitarianism, 121, 177

Virtue ethics, 121, 177

Whistleblowing, 101, 103, 181